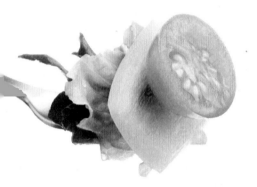

High Raw

A Simple Approach to Health, Eating, and Saving the Planet

BY
KEVIN GIANNI

WWW.GOHIGHRAW.COM

RHTV

First Edition
Edited by Heather Fougnier
Cover Design and Layout by Tara Mayberry, AugustDesignStudio.com

A Better Life Press
P.O. Box 228
Bethel, CT 06801

Gianni, Kevin M.
High Raw : a simple approach to health, eating and
saving the planet / by Kevin Gianni. – 1st ed.
p. cm.
Includes bibliographical references and index.
LCCN 2008912095
ISBN-13: 978-0-9788123-4-8
ISBN-10: 0-9788123-4-4

1. Raw food diet. 2. Nutrition. 3. Health.
I. Title.

RM237.5.G53 2009 613.2'6
QBI09-200026

PRINTED IN THE USA

www.GoHighRaw.com and www.RenegadeHealth.com

Medical Warning and Disclaimer

The information in this book is not intended as medical advice or to replace a one-on-one relationship with a qualified health care professional. It is intended as a sharing of knowledge and information from the research and experience of Kevin Gianni. We encourage you to make your own health care decisions based upon your research and in partnership with a qualified health care professional.

This book is printed on 100% post-consumer recycled paper, manufactured chlorine free, with vegetable-based inks, using new environmental technology by **seedsgreenprinting.com**

10 trees preserved for the future	4,192 gal wastewater flow saved	464 lbs solid waste not generated	564 lbs net greenhouse gases prevented	6,990,400 BTUs energy not consumed

Review your reusing and recycling practices and invest in our future!

FOREWORD

When Kevin asked me to write the foreword for his new book, *High Raw*, I was delighted. I've had the honor and privilege of working with him on many occasions and know him to be "the real deal." He is one of the best motivators around— whether you're working with him in person, listening to or viewing his online programs, or reading his books. As you can probably tell, I am one of his biggest fans.

Every page of this book inspires me. I use it as part of the arsenal of information I bring to my clients and students as they start in their journey of physical self-awareness and optimum health. This journey is not just one of left-brained evaluation, or simply one of judging fitness or lack-of-dis-ease levels. This is a journey of discovering the reader's own potential for health. Kevin's uplifting book sincerely, and very practically, helps each reader evaluate their current level of health, and create the essential mind-set for making very deep and lasting changes in their lives. High Raw is a superlative guide that will take you on a thrilling process of uncovering your potential in every area of your life.

The process of simply reading this book will move your unconscious mind towards a new base of knowledge of your body and health. This new place will give you the grounding and clarity to help sort out the confusing messages coming from your normal sources of health information. Kevin's writing comes from the heart and from the standpoint of a journalist. He shares what he has witnessed and experienced in his own journey from lethargy and complete unawareness of his own health, to a place of feeling consistent motivation and inspiration and high physical energy levels, which is the real goal of improving our health.

It seems that the current state of most modern societies is one of frantic unawareness. Fast, "busyness," focus on work and money, and unrealistic expectations are perfect descriptions, and the gaps usually filled in with mind-numbing entertainment, all of which ensures that we will never have the time, energy, or space to create the self-knowledge we need to truly care for our bodies. Very few parents, schools, TV shows, websites, medical institutions, or other common sources of information, are conveying a message of finding a true sense of fulfillment. Unfortunately, and too often, for many people, the moments they realize that there is truly more in life than what they've experienced is something that is shocking and profound.

These same sources of information are usually the source of our health information, or rather lack of health information. If they aren't conveying a message that helps us live to our fullest potential and strive to ensure that others can do the same, then they aren't conveying a message of true health. If we are to be aware of our health on every level, we need to be truly motivated. This motivation factor is what Kevin does best. When our mind can wrap itself around these concepts, it can then help to make real, and lasting, changes in our lives.

I particularly like Kevin's superb book title, High Raw. On

his health journey, Kevin found that optimum health begins by eating a whole foods-based diet of mostly vegetables, fruits, nuts, seeds. He also understands, as a rapidly growing number of people throughout this country now realize, too, that this way of eating is the quickest way to make positive changes in our physical and emotional health. He encourages readers to "think like a raw food vegan." In his easygoing, reader-friendly, and non-judgmental manner, Kevin suggests that we create meals based largely on fresh, colorful plant-based foods: vegetables, fruits, nuts, and seeds for at least two weeks, and see what changes this makes in our energy levels. Additionally, he suggests that we all "lighten up." Put simply, don't be too strict or hard on ourselves; this only sets up the potential for failure, which is the last thing that any of us need, right?

For the past 30 years, in my own private practice, magazine articles and interviews, and in my workshops and holistic retreats worldwide, I encourage everyone to live a holistic lifestyle. This means to live healthfully in body, mind, and spirit and make vibrant health a way of life. To do this, we must incorporate the following: embrace a natural-foods diet; get enough sleep; use natural remedies; exercise frequently; detoxify and rejuvenate often; drink ample purified water; keep stress levels down; spend time in nature; breathe deeply and meditate; and cultivate an attitude of gratitude. Kevin concurs with me on all of these tenets necessary for optimum health. If we want to live with high energy, vibrancy and a celebration for life, we must choose to make changes now. No one can do it for you. You must first decide to make health your top priority and move in that direction, with Kevin's help and expertise. And to make this change, an easy-to-follow roadmap is key to a path of least resistance. Kevin's empowering book will help you start fresh, with no judgment, and provides all the tools and information necessary for you to be successful.

It's also refreshing for me to see a young messenger like Kevin, a shining example of healthy living, spread this inspiring message, instead of one promoting gadgets, fad foods and fly-by-night ideas like many health authors do. We all need a little help from our friends. Invite Kevin (and *High Raw*) to be your friend in your journey to experience vibrant health in body, mind and spirit. If you do, you will achieve your goals, create your best life, and thank your lucky stars that you have Kevin as your guide.

— Susan Smith Jones, PhD, author of *Health Bliss, The Healing Power of NatureFoods, Be Healthy— Stay Balanced and Recipes for Health Bliss*: www.SusanSmithJones.com

TABLE OF CONTENTS

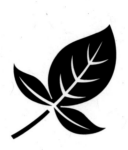

A NEW PARADIGM FOR HEALTH

Today, we have access to more health information and scientific studies than ever before and yet, two things are happening:

(1) There is more confusion than ever about what is healthy.

(2) Health epidemics like diabetes, heart disease, food allergies, cancer and obesity are on the rise.

Why is this happening?

TOO MANY PEOPLE ARE CONFUSED ABOUT HEALTH

Nearly half of all American adults — 90 million people — have difficulty understanding and acting upon health information.

—INSTITUTE OF MEDICINE REPORT: HEALTH LITERACY:
A PRESCRIPTION TO END CONFUSION (2004).

Americans give media health reports low trust and credibility ratings, and almost as many say media health reports confuse them as say they provide useful information.

—GALLUP NEWS SERVICE FROM 2002 GALLUP POLL

It's time to demystify health and how YOU can get and STAY healthy. I wrote *High Raw* because I want to give you information that is straight to the point and laid back. No ego, no fancy promises and nothing overwhelming.

The idea of *"High Raw"* is by no means new. Many people have been eating a diet of ripe fruits and vegetables for thousands of years.

What's different about what you're about to read is that I've simplified the process of creating your best health with raw foods. Probably even more than anyone else I've learned from.

Why? Because I want you to actually succeed. I want to make it easy for you.

I've stripped away my ego to bring you the simplest and most valuable information in the shortest amount of time. There won't be any lengthy scientific arguments here. For those you can go somewhere else and get even more confused. I'll cover this in chapter 2.

For as you and I both know, if there's a scientific study for something, anyone can find the complete opposite finding somewhere else.

In *High Raw*, I'm including what works. Here, you'll find shortcuts to the best of eight to ten years of my own personal journey, including my study of fitness and nutrition from hundreds of books, articles and interviews with top experts.

High Raw is about much more than what to eat or how to eat it. We'll go way beyond that and address creating a foundation of health, listening to your body and your intuition and building a toolbox with strategies to get started and maintain your best health. And if you haven't gotten to know me yet through my blog, RenegadeHealth.com, you'll find out quickly that I want you to have fun along the way!

When you think of good health, what comes to mind?
Instead of thinking of complicated answers about heart health, Body Mass Index, fitness and diet foods, what about just a simple statement…good health is really about feeling your best, isn't it?

The key to feeling your best is not a complex equation and it doesn't require pouring over the latest statistics from journals full of medical mumbo jumbo. In fact, achieving your best health can be quite easy — and that's the goal of *High Raw* — cutting through the confusion and keeping it simple.

If you're like me, you're busy…you've had enough of the back and forth about the latest health fads that are here today and debunked tomorrow. You just want to feel good… and you want to have fun while doing it!

It is my mission to introduce a new paradigm for health, a paradigm where feeling your best is simple. Where we leave out the mystery and embrace a common sense approach to feeling energized, fit, happy and healthy.

In the old paradigm, good health was confusing, overwhelming and downright boring. *High Raw* introduces a new paradigm for health: where you become empowered to use your own intuition and take small steps with powerful tools to feel your best. The most important part? Have fun! Good health is a journey and you deserve to smile and enjoy the trip!

OLD PARADIGM	NEW PARADIGM
Latest health fads	Back to basics and common sense approaches
Confusing and conflicting information	Educating yourself with simple principles and tools
Relying on medicine for health	Relying on simple good habits for health

OLD PARADIGM	NEW PARADIGM
Feeling overwhelmed with complex systems	Taking small steps and using helpful tools
Dull, boring and difficult choices	Fun, motivating and simple choices

YOUR ADVENTURE IN HEALTH

So what if creating your best health was a great adventure?

Let's take a wild ride and enjoy this trip together! But before we officially take off on this adventure, I want to finish up this introduction with a possibility...

Imagine if you could just enjoy your food...without guilt, without shame, without questioning.

It's possible — and some of the answers are right here in this book.

The fact is that the answers to healthy eating are right in front of us. We've just chosen to ignore them. Not because we want to ignore them, but because we're surrounded by messages that make this exploration of health into something much harder than it is. But no matter what the media or scientific studies tell you, good health is NOT as complicated as programming a super computer. In reality, it can be as simple as flipping a switch.

I have a laminated sheet with a few of my goals that I pin up in the shower. (Yes, the shower!) On it is this saying, which my good friend, Jonathan, shared with me:

> *If someone taught me how to flip a switch,*
> *I wouldn't spend any time wondering how it*
> *worked, I'd just enjoy the light.*

Let's start enjoying the light. Let's keep our mind open to possibilities. When we do, we'll find the answers.

That's what this book is about.

A LITTLE ABOUT ME (OR IF I CAN DO IT, SO CAN YOU!)

Seriously...I was not the paragon of good health. I had some pretty terrible habits that I didn't really feel the need to do anything about — until my physical and emotional health started to suffer.

Let's start with high school. To begin with, I was an athlete, playing football, basketball and tennis. As co-captain of my football team, I celebrated winning the 1995 Connecticut State Football Championship. In tennis, I was on the top doubles team in the conference.

So I always understood that fitness was very important, in fact, I still think it's one of the most important things you can do.

Anyway, my fitness was taken care of in high school. I knew how to weight-lift, albeit the wrong way, but still, I knew how to build muscle. I knew how to exercise and I knew how to compete and be competitive in sports.

What I didn't know anything about was nutrition. Absolutely nothing.

In fact, my tennis doubles partner and I had what we thought was great energy food before a match. We'd go to the school store, this little hole in the wall that was always full of candy, soda and other processed foods. We'd each pick out a package of Twinkies and a can of Mountain Dew.

To add insult to injury, after our little "energizing snack," we'd jump into my mother's Dodge Caravan, drive to a spot in the neighborhood behind the school, and smoke a cigarette. Then we would come back and park by the tennis courts and start our tennis match.

So that was my nutritional background...Not so hot, huh?

Well, things didn't get much better in college.

When I got into college I decided not to pursue any sports.

Instead, like many other students, I became adept at the art of partying. I became a self-proclaimed, beer-slugging loser.

I partied all the time. And it didn't help that I was going to college in the state of New York, where bars stay open until 4:00 in the morning! My friends and I must have thought that just because the bars were open, we had to be there, because we'd play pool, drink and hang out until closing.

For a while, it seemed like the be-all end-all of fun. But over time, it really wore on me. I would wake up at two in the afternoon, go to class (well, if I even wanted to go to class!) and I even kept up with my workout routine.

Eventually, I began to gain weight, despite all of the time I spent in the gym. Over time, I gained thirty pounds. I felt overweight, lazy and tired. Truthfully, I was unhappy and uncomfortable with myself. I felt I had lost my drive and my focus.

I couldn't think what to do with my life, except to go out the next night and party as usual. My lifestyle became vicious cycle that played out, literally, for the entire four years of college.

After college, the partying continued and my life seemed to get even worse. To get the full effect, you have to picture how I lived: imagine a basement apartment in Brooklyn, NY. I shared this tiny space with a friend, who I was working with at the time.

The place was so small, that I had a makeshift room created by stringing a sheet between my bed and the rest of the apartment. Every day, I'd get up, walk around the sheet and sit at my desk doing web design projects. At night, I'd be out partying as usual. It wasn't long before all of the good things seemed to drain out of my life, between sitting in that basement and partying too late into the night. My relationships suffered, from my roommate to my family to my friends. I became miserable and found myself sinking into depression.

One night, after a particularly late night of drunken partying, I came home and slept until two o'clock the next afternoon. If you've ever peeled your head off the pillow after too much alcohol, you can imagine how I felt that day.

My head was spinning, I felt awful and something inside me shifted. It was in this moment that I asked myself a question: "Is there something better than this?"

That one question changed my life.

Because the answer was the kind of positive kick in the butt that made me take action in a better direction.

That very day, I got my head straight, called my mother and told her I was moving home. I admitted that I couldn't work or live like this anymore. My mother said, "You can move home and stay in the guestroom, but you can't put any of your clothes in the dresser." That was fine with me, because I knew it was a starting point for change. I told my friend that I was quitting my job and moved back home. With that one act, doors started to open for me.

One of the doors that opened came when my mother handed me a book. The book was called *The Seeker's Guide* by Elizabeth Lesser, who was the co-founder of Omega Institute.

Before that time, I was never open to the idea or the possibility that maybe there was more to life — and more to health — than just fitness. I hadn't really thought much about things like spirituality and nutrition. *The Seeker's Guide* opened my mind to the possibility that there was so much more than I was already experiencing.

That possibility has led to where I am right now. That one grain of possibility allowed me to go from feeling lazy, tired, anxious, angry, depressed and stressed out to feeling happy, optimistic and passionate about my life and work. Don't get me wrong, I still have challenges and I still get stressed out at times (you can ask my wife and business partner, Annmarie, about that!), but since that day, I created a whole new foundation for how I live my life.

I share my experience to show you that no matter how bad things look, you can start with one question, one book, one inspiration and transform your life! All you have to do is be ready.

So if you're ready, I'd like to share some information, tools and strategies that can kick start your own transformation. If you're ready, this book may be the one thing that changes your life for the better!

CHAPTER 1

HOW DID WE GET SO OFF TRACK WITH DIET AND HEALTH?

Somehow, we got off track when it comes to health. You may have heard media reports saying that we are living longer than ever, but are we living better?

Obesity, diabetes, heart disease, allergies, asthma, ADD, autism and other health issues are on the rise...and not just for adults. These conditions are affecting kids too. Illnesses that confound doctors, like chronic fatigue, fibromyalgia and candida are causing thousands of people to suffer.

According to the World Health Organization, one of the growing concerns worldwide is chronic and non-communicable diseases like diabetes, cardiovascular disease, depression and cancers.[1] Non-communicable diseases are those that are not infectious and can result from genetic or lifestyle factors. They tend to develop over long periods of time, often without symptoms at first.

So while statistics may show we are living longer, we are not necessarily living better.

Sally Fallon, author of the book, *Nourishing Traditions*, wrote an article comparing our quality of life with that of our ancestors.

Sally Fallon argues that our lives are actually not better today then they were in past generations. If you look around, you'd probably agree with her findings: too many people today suffer from "degenerative diseases — arthritis, multiple sclerosis, digestive disorders, diabetes, osteoporosis, Alzheimer's, epilepsy and chronic fatigue...Learning disabilities such as dyslexia and hyperactivity make life miserable for seven million young people — not to mention their parents."[2]

HOW DID WE GET SO OFF TRACK?

When did we decide that medical technology and over-the-counter and prescription drugs were the answers to help us live healthier and longer?

Are we relying on something outside of ourselves, like doctors and medicine, to keep us healthy, when in fact, we may hold the greatest key of all to our health and longevity? Before we examine that, let's take a look at just how successful medicine is at keeping us healthy.

In his book, *Death by Medicine*, Gary Null has gathered statistics to show that modern medicine may actually be harmful to your health! We all know that the American health care system is a mess, but it hits home when you learn some of the statistics Gary Null shares about accidental deaths, unnecessary hospitalizations, unnecessary prescriptions (for antibiotics, especially) and unnecessary surgeries.

Here are some statistics of a medical system gone awry from *Death by Medicine*[3].

Adverse Drug Reactions in Hospitals	106,000 Deaths Annually
Medical Errors	98,000 Deaths Annually
Unnecessary Procedures	37,136 Deaths Annually

The cost of these three medical interventions alone is approximately $136,000,000 annually. Literally billions of dollars spent on medical errors. But it gets worse.

According to Null, when you add up all of the medical and drug errors across all categories, it is estimated at 999,936 deaths annually, which amounts to 7.8 million deaths over 10 years of medical intervention.[4]

Something is wrong with this picture. We may be living longer, but the very system we are relying on to keep us healthy is broken. This is not to say that doctors and medical interventions don't save lives, but the idea that we'd willingly hand over responsibility for our health to a system that is plagued with problems is one of the reasons we've gotten off track.

The good news is that more and more people are taking responsibility for their own health. Just the fact that you are reading this book tells me that you are one of them and I acknowledge you for that!

So what does it take to be self-responsible when it comes to your own health? I'll cover the specifics in the upcoming chapters of this book. But first, I want to talk about creating a mindset for good health.

The first step in creating a mindset for good health is believing that YOU are in charge of your own best health. Once you become aware of that, the rest gets easier.

I always recommend that you work with a qualified health practitioner. Who you choose is up to you. But when you recognize that YOU are responsible for your health, you become part of the process of creating your health. Instead of giving up control to someone else, you become a partner with your health practitioner. This means that you'll have actions to take to change your health picture. You'll find many excellent tools here in this book to support you. The good news is that when you start taking action, you become empowered to feel your best. You are no longer a victim when you realize that the habits you create and the lifestyle you lead holds the key to your health.

When you choose to take action and start to create a lifestyle that supports good health, some of the things you may change are: the foods you eat, how much exercise you do and how much stress you have in your life.

The Centers for Disease Control and Prevention (CDC) states that up to 90% of doctor's visits may be triggered by stress-related illness.[5]

Many natural health experts agree that chronic stress causes is at the heart of most of our emotional and physical health conditions today. Why are so many people feeling so stressed out?

I used to feel the negative effects of chronic stress myself and much of it has to do with taking a good look at how you are living your life. Chapters 10 and 11 of this book are full of tools and strategies to help you create a foundation for success and make your healthy habits stick.

It's important to remember that taking action for your health is important, but if you get too stressed out about our health, it can have adverse affects.

The truth is that there's a lot of conflicting and confusing information in the media, scientific studies and from health and medical experts. I'll tell you why this is happening in chapter 2. If you get too stressed out about it, you'll end up worrying and forget to enjoy the journey. Chapters three and four will guide you toward ways to cut through all the confusion about health information and find out what really works for you.

Good health doesn't have to be hard. So if you find yourself feeling confused and frustrated, take a deep breath, and review chapters 4–9, where I outline some simple, common sense principles for diet and health.

CHAPTER 2

SCIENCE, MEDICINE, AND MEDIA — WHAT CAN YOU REALLY BELIEVE?

With more availability of information about health than ever before, why are we still so confused? Why are chronic health conditions still on the rise?

Let's stop and think for a moment about the SOURCE of where this health information is coming from. The major sources are: scientific studies, medicine (doctors, pharmaceutical companies) and the media (television, newspapers, journals). It's important that you understand how these sources of information can be biased, before you decide what to believe.

SCIENCE — DO WE NEED IT? IS IT VALUABLE?

I have a love/hate relationship with science. On the one hand, I have a scientific mindset. I love to read studies and look at data. I believe in getting baseline tests when it comes to your health. And I believe that we have to go through processes and systems in order to really decide if something's working or not — whether we're talking about your body or even machines, like your car or appliances, like your toaster oven.

The American Heritage Dictionary defines science as "Knowledge, especially that gained through experience" and "The observation, identification, description, experimental investigation, and theoretical explanation of phenomena."

Experimenting with what works and coming up with systems is helpful. For example, if you were building a house, you'd find out all the tools, materials, people and steps you needed to make it work. You might experiment a bit as you are learning to build the house and once you build your first one, you could replicate that process when you build another house. You'd have a system...that's a type of science.

You probably do the same thing in many areas of your life. At work, you've found systems and processes that help you get your job done. At home, you have routines and processes for your life, like what time you eat your meals. That's actually a scientific process and these can be really helpful to us. But it's not like all that science gobbledy-gook that can be so confusing, like chemical formulas.

Here's the deal, when it comes to our nutrition, I think science has gone horribly wrong. Some people will argue till their death about that with me, but I've seen too many people confused and it's time to expose this truth.

First of all, nutrition science has not been around that long. In Michael Pollan's book, *In Defense of Food: An Eater's Manifesto Manifesto*, he likens nutrition science to surgery in 1650, "which is to say very interesting and promising, but do you really want to get on the table yet?"[1] Back then, it was only just beginning and people didn't know much about it. With nutrition science, it's been around for only 175 years and today, we still don't know everything there is to know. One day fat is bad for you and the next, we learn there is good fat. So after years of eating fat free diets, many people started experiencing health issues like depression, from lack of good fats. Then it was all about low carb/no carb/high protein and it seems to continue with new things popping up each year. Over the past 175 years, nutrition science has been rife with fads and conflicting information. No wonder so many people are confused!

Here are a few reasons to question science:

- REASON #1: WE ARE MORE THAN THE SUM OF OUR PARTS

  I really believe that science is breaking things down into too many pieces and taking a reductionist approach. The reductionist approach breaks things down to the smallest pieces and observes them to make theories about the whole. While this can be useful in many ways, the danger is that if we forget the whole, we can make big mistakes when it comes to health.

  It's like treating a disease, but not looking at how the treatment will affect the whole person. We are complex beings. We are not just one cell or one organ. If you treat the one cell or one organ, without thinking about how it affects the whole person, you could be doing more harm than good.

  The same is true in nutrition science. Foods are broken down to their smallest parts, like beta carotene, lycopene or essential fatty acids. Scientists look at those small parts and make recommendations about what they do for our bodies. The next thing you know, all the manufactured foods add these ingredients in or supplements are made to give us those amazing ingredients. How do we know that those ingredients alone, when extracted from the

> With nutrition science, it's been around for only 175 years and today, we still don't know everything there is to know... Over the past 175 years, nutrition science has been rife with fads and conflicting information. No wonder so many people are confused!

fruits and vegetables they came from are doing what they are supposed to do? This is Michael Pollan's argument in his book, *In Defense of Food*. He contends that we may be better off simply sticking to fruits and vegetables because we know they work.[2]

- **REASON #2: MONEY TALKS: THE SWAYING OF SCIENCE, NUTRITION & HEALTH**

Did you know that scientific studies are often swayed by those who fund them? A big question we should all be asking is "where did the money originate to fund a scientific study?"

Unfortunately, the big money to fund scientific studies often comes from the drug companies.

Studies are funded by pharmaceutical companies and conducted by medical experts. But when it comes to presenting results, the pharmaceutical staff often works with scientists to determine how the results should be presented. This has led to abuses, like study results being omitted if results did not show a product in a favorable light.[3]

In 2001, the *International Committee of Medical Journal Editors'*, which includes prestigious journals such as the *Journal of the American Medical Association (JAMA)* and the *New England Journal of Medicine (NEJM)*, created a new policy refusing to publish studies unless researchers were guaranteed scientific independence.[4]

But that didn't fix the problem because in 2004, Center for Science in the Public Interest exposed *JAMA* and other journals for publishing scientific studies without disclosing who paid for the studies.[5]

> Did you know that scientific studies are often swayed by those who fund them? A big question we should all be asking is "where did the money originate to fund a scientific study?"

Too many of these scientific studies are being published to dupe the public into making conclusions about the benefits of certain products, namely, pharmaceutical drugs. And it doesn't stop with scientific studies. You can follow the money trail right to your doctor's office, because they too, are being swayed by money from pharmaceutical and biomedical companies.

In fact, in 2006, the *Boston Globe* reported that Stanford medical center joined several other well-known academic medical centers in a new policy that would allow their research to be independent of drug companies. As public knowledge of tainted research practices escalated, these academic medical centers recognized that conflicts of interest had the potential to influence how they trained staff and provided clinical care. According to the *Boston Globe*, "Of the $21 billion the pharmaceutical industry spends every year on marketing, as much as 90 percent is directed at physicians through various mechanisms, such as free meals, gifts and drug samples and sponsorship of continuing medical education programs and other events..."[6]

So while most of us have been led to believe we can trust doctors, you have to question them too. Doctors, medical school education and studies are all subject to potential conflicts of interest from drug companies. This is not to say that there aren't great doctors and health care practitioners out there. But it might surprise you to find out that most doctors think the majority of their peers are swayed by the influence of money from drug companies.[7]

Keep in mind that it's not just pharmaceutical and biomedical companies that have money to sway science. From big agribusiness industries like dairy, corn and beef to personal care products and baby products, big money is spent to lobby the US Congress or the FDA to sway decisions in their favor. These decisions result in recommendations as to what we should eat and how safe our food and personal care products are.

Recently, Bristol-Myers Squibb, a New York based pharmaceutical spent $840,000 lobbying Congress on the safety of Bisphenol A (a known toxin) used in its baby formula food packaging.[8] And Monsanto, one of the largest agribusiness companies, funded a group of farmers lobbying for the right to use synthetic bovine growth hormone (a product made by Monsanto) for increased milk production.[9]

The truth of it is this: the lettuce lobby is not on the steps of Washington fighting for red leaf lettuce. There's no one fighting for kale. There's no one fighting for grapes or raisins. The people who are fighting are people who have vested interests, like the supplement companies, big agribusiness, large manufactured food companies and the pharmaceuticals. Their intentions are (as you can guess) to get research out there that supports their cause or to fight the research that was against their product.

This is why there is so much conflicting and confusing information when it comes to health and nutrition. You can look up any scientific study and find the complete opposite for it. It's because this sort of jockeying is happening all the time.

While there may be plenty of altruistic people who want to go to the government or into the school systems to really get people healthy—with no biased agenda—they simply don't have the kind of financial backing that the large industries have.

There's no money fight for lettuce because it's just not

that large of an industry. Corn, wheat, dairy, beef, pork, all these other conglomerates are fighting to get their products known. This has been going on for years. The generations before us, particularly between 1930 and 1970, were influenced by these industries, which is why they are so set on the paradigm of meat and dairy.

Dairy lobbies and meat lobbies influenced everything from the messages about how much of their products to consume to even the food pyramid recommended by US dieticians! Insider Marion Nestle, chair of New York University's Department of Nutrition and Food Studies and author of *Food Politics: How the Food Industry Influences Nutrition, and Health*, details just how lobbyists influence the food pyramid, product sales through lobbying, financial contributions, lawsuits, public relations, alliances and other tactics.

According to statistics from the Humane Society, the amount of meat consumption has increased 154 percent from 1950 to 2007.[10] Based on what you've learned about lobbyists, that may not seem like a surprise. The other reason for an increase in meat eating is that as people become more affluent, they eat more in general, including an increase in meat consumption. Lester R. Brown, author of *Plan B 3.0: Mobilizing to Save Civilization*, wrote about this phenomenon, stating that the poor are concerned about too little to eat and the rich are concerned about eating too much. In fact, this has been influenced in the types of disease experienced by these economic groups. In *Plan B*, Brown writes that the 1.2 billion wealthiest people in the world are dying of diseases of aging and excessive lifestyle, like obesity, smoking, high fat and high sugar diets and lack of exercise.[11]

In contrast, the 1.2 billion poorest people are dying

from infectious diseases and malnutrition. Brown contends that since the poorest populations are malnourished from eating too low on the food chain and the richest populations experience disease from eating too high on the food chain, the best solution is to eat in the middle of the food chain. This means more of a largely plant-based diet, with a smaller amount of meat and grains.[12]

So if you look at that, that's where today's nutrition paradigm is. The rich were eating meat. When talking to my grandfather and my mother, they felt like eating steak meant they were eating like kings. You may have experienced this as well. In some families eating steak regularly is too expensive. While I personally don't eat meat, I'm not against it. I know that it has a place for some people in their diet. But when you look at how meat lobbyists have influenced our consumption, you have to stop and think about what's really the right amount for your best health.

The lobbyists for all these companies are always out working. *Appetite for Profit*, by Michele Simon, is another book that exposes tactics used by lobbyists for companies like Coca-Cola, McDonalds and Kraft to make their foods seem healthier than they really are. In *Appetite for Profit*, Simon also focuses on how children are targets for many of these company campaigns. For example, in a conflict with mothers about selling soda in school, compromises were reached to continue selling soda, as long as it wasn't during the school day. The scary part is that because they have the financial backing, they are winning. And they don't have our best interest or children's best interest at heart.

Money talks, so when it comes to information about

health and nutrition, stay alert to where the information is coming from. Chapter 8 will cover more about how to educate yourself and cut through all of the conflicting information that is out there.

- **REASON #3: A SIGNIFICANT PERCENTAGE OF RESEARCH IS FLAWED**

Imagine building a house on a crumbling foundation. You might build the best house, but over time, as the foundation crumbles, the structure of the house will break and crumble as well.

Now let's apply that to science. Many scientific studies are built upon previous studies...but what happens if the previous studies were flawed? All medical research goes through a "peer review," which is essentially a review of each study by a group of scientists and experts who are supposed to be unbiased.

When the studies pass the peer review process, people often take action based on those studies. Doctors may prescribe drugs or protocols based on them, which means you may be affected by the study results.

In 2005, serious flaws were exposed in the peer review process. In fact, "almost one-third of top research articles over the 10-year period studied, have been either contradicted or seriously questioned," according to an article in the *Boston Globe*.[13] These studies had created a decade of recommendations and further studies that affected our health.

If you consider one study a foundation for further studies, imagine how much incorrect information is influencing us? If science keeps building on a faulty foundation, eventually, just like the house, it will topple.

Advertisements today are riddled with magic bullets and quick fixes to any problem you might have. But don't be fooled, these slick, high budget, weapons of mass influence are targeted at reaching their desired goal, regardless of your best interests.

MEDIA INFLUENCE — ADS, ENDORSEMENTS AND MIRACLE FIXES

It's not just science that influences what we think about nutrition, the media plays a tremendous role in what and how we eat, including our thoughts about food. As much as we hate to admit it, the media does influence us.

A 2002 Gallup poll showed that the amount of time the media has focused on health has grown. Because "health sells," television, magazines, newspapers and the Internet have all started devoting more "air time" to health and nutrition. This has not, however, helped people understand nutrition any better, nor do people trust health media, according to Gallup.[14]

Is it possible to trust the media's portrayal of health and nutrition?

Here are some reasons why so many people don't trust the media:

- REASON #1: ADVERTISEMENTS — THE GREAT MADISON AVENUE DECEPTION

  Marketing is a science in and of itself. It's the science of influencing people that they have a problem that a certain product or service can solve. First, if the problem is well known, like being overweight, it's probably pretty easy to sell a solution. But marketing techniques go deeper than that. They also aim to educate you about problems you don't even know you have! A great deal of money is spent simply on marketing, to get you to think you have a problem and need to buy something to solve it.

  When it comes to food, much of the advertising

budgets are aimed at getting you to want a certain food…and when they aren't selling enough of that food, they aim to get you to want to eat more of that food. Remember the fat free craze of the 90's, when it seemed okay to eat more of something because it was "fat free?" A great deal of research and psychology goes into advertisements and whether we want to admit it or not, they can influence us.

Advertisements today are riddled with magic bullets and quick fixes to any problem you might have. But don't be fooled, these slick, high budget, weapons of mass influence are targeted at reaching their desired goal, regardless of your best interests.

According to a study in The Journal of Health Communication, from 1996 to 2000, drug ads aimed at consumers has more than tripled, with the highest percentage spent on television ads.[15] The study showed that an average TV watcher was exposed to more drug ads than any other form of health information.

What I find interesting is that you also see TV ads from Mothers Against Drunk Driving telling people how awful drunk driving is, but yet, there are even more ads on TV from pharmaceuticals, that kill far more people than drunk drivers. Drunk driving caused 13,407 fatalities in 2006.[16] In *Death by Medicine*, Gary Null's data from 1994 showed that 106,000 deaths occurred annually from adverse drug reactions in hospitals and the numbers are growing.[17]

- REASON #2: PRESS RELEASES — FANCY ADS DESIGNED TO LOOK LIKE FACTS
Press releases are written to provide compelling information and a call to action that looks and feels like a newspaper or magazine article. There are also video news

releases, which are produced with the same goal for TV news. With shrinking budgets and resources, too many reporters are cutting corners and engaging in the practice of using press releases verbatim or in essence, plagiarizing large pieces of a press release and making it look like real journalism. Science, health and medical journalism has been hard-hit by this practice and according to some experts, it's getting worse with the proliferation of digital news on the Internet.[18]

Papers can be literally from 50–70 percent direct press releases from a specific company. Who's writing the press releases? Companies and people who want to get their specific message out.

Last year, I was speaking to an audience of about 40 people at Iona College in New Rochelle, NY. I asked the audience, "Does anyone work for the school paper?" One girl raised her hand. I said, "Let me ask you a question. Do you get press releases?" She said, "Yes." I said, "What do you do with them?" She replied, "Well, we decide which ones we want to print in the paper." When I asked her if she rewrote the press releases, she said, "No. We just publish them." Now that's a college paper, but don't think that that practice doesn't move up the ladder. It's a lazy way of journalism, but it's also a way to fill paper. It's a way to get information out there. The problem is that press releases are biased and they are often passed off as a good, objective journalistic article.

There was a study that came out in 2005 and the headline in Fox News was: "Study: Coffee Top Source of Antioxidants."[19] There were huge headlines, all over the place — this was big stuff. People were emailing me asking, "Kevin did you see this? Coffee is a good source of antioxidants." Well guess what happened? The journalist made a mistake; they didn't read the full study. Do you know what the full study said? It said this: "Coffee is the highest source of America's antioxidants." It did not say coffee was a good source of antioxidants. It said that coffee is where Americans get most of their antioxidants. This is plain inaccurate. Coffee is by far NOT one of the best sources of antioxidants. For example, blueberries are giants in terms of antioxidant content when compared to coffee.

- REASON #3: ENDORSEMENTS — USING CELEBRITIES AND EXPERTS TO GAIN YOUR TRUST
In marketing, endorsements are another technique to sell products and services. The idea is to pay an expert, athlete or celebrity, someone you'd trust or admire, to recommend their product. Endorsements are being used more and more often in all kinds of marketing from advertisements to television and magazine articles. You'll even see a growing number of endorsements on the Internet.

There are many people profiting from endorsements, so be aware of whom you decide to trust. The good news is, there are a growing number of people out there who have high integrity and would only recommend what has been successful in their own lives. You'll know the difference the more you stay alert for the messages you are watching, reading or hearing.

BECOMING YOUR OWN DETECTIVE

So let's be careful. We can't just look at these studies and just think that this information is right. We have to be detectives. I like to tell people that we can be our own "scientific research labs." Everybody laughs when I say this, but it's true. That's what I've done with myself. Sometimes you mess up and sometimes you really succeed. Or you have to reach out to people who you know are really walking their talk — the people you trust or the people you know. Have a smart mind around it.

In chapter 7, I will actually take you through a process — a scientific process of getting results. If you were to take one simple process that I use myself and teach to others, you will more easily determine what works for you. You'll learn to know and trust your own body and your own intuition. This is what will make the already easy principles of *High Raw* even easier! And it will make your journey through the jungle of nutrition and health information seem like a fun adventure. So you can relax and enjoy the ride.

CHAPTER 3

HIGH RAW: A SIMPLE SOLUTION FOR DIET AND HEALTH

CUTTING THROUGH THE CONFUSION

So how did I go from a "beer slugging loser with Brooklyn Basement-itis" to a successful, happy entrepreneur? I went on a personal quest to find answers. For years, I've been researching natural health, healing, fitness, self-development and nutrition; and interviewing some of the top experts in the field.

And what I found was this...conflicting information, complex systems, and downright confusion. Now that you've read chapters 1 and 2, you understand why.

When it comes to nutrition, I think of myself as a journalist. And as a journalist, there's one thing I know for sure: it's time to breakdown the stiff and cold nutritional guidelines, calorie counting diets and charts and re-learn the tenets of health that create lasting results.

First of all, let's start with some basic common sense that just about everyone can agree upon when it comes to nutrition:

- EAT AS CLOSE TO NATURE AS POSSIBLE: like whole fresh fruits, vegetables, nuts and seeds

- EAT LESS PROCESSED FOODS (better yet, eliminate processed foods entirely!)

When it comes to healthy eating, I am certainly an advocate of eating more raw food. The raw food movement is growing and many people are catching on to its simple message. And yet, what should be simple is actually becoming complicated by a lot of conflicting diet and nutrition information.

Why? Because everyone is looking for scientific proof and as you've already seen from the previous chapters, this can be a slippery slope.

I experienced this first hand after I started my own blog TV show, "The Renegade Health Show," also known as rhTV. The goal of "The Renegade Health" show, which you can watch at www.RenegadeHealth.com, is to provide a fun, exciting, easy-to-understand and educational forum for natural health enthusiasts.

Each month, tens of thousands of viewers in over 85 countries tune into "The Renegade Health Show," so you can imagine that I get a lot of questions about diet, nutrition, exercise and raw foods.

Here are some very common questions I receive about the raw food diet:

- "I hear such conflicting information about optimum health from a raw food perspective. How can I do this?"

- "Do I have to be 100 percent raw?"

- "What foods will enhance what I'm doing?"

- "What foods will help me heal?"

The truth is, while you'd think the premise of eating raw food would be easy, the raw food diet can be just as complex as any other dietary program. I've seen completely opposing viewpoints in discussions on my Inner Circle, where over a thousand members discuss natural health, with guidance from thought leaders and experts.

If you look anywhere across the board: the Internet, books, radio, TV, videos on YouTube or online, you're going to be able to find exactly the opposite information to what you want to find. You're going to end up finding things at complete different ends of the spectrum.

It's time to cut through the confusion. This is where *High Raw* comes in. *High Raw* honors the fact that we all want easy to follow information that we can use to suit our unique situations. And of course, we want to enjoy the journey, so it should be fun!

The principle behind *High Raw* is to filter the information on raw food and nutrition and break it down to the common sense principles that really matter. So you can wipe out the confusion and wipe out the feelings of shame or guilt when it comes to your diet. Imagine how that would feel.... Imagine if by the end of this book, you could say, "Wow. I really believe this is easy. I can do this."

So let's talk about the concept of *"High Raw"* and what that means with respect to the raw food diet and nutrition as a whole.

WHAT IS HIGH RAW?

The raw food diet is based on whole, organic, uncooked, unprocessed fruits, vegetables, nuts, seeds, beans and seaweeds. Much of the raw food movement focuses on a largely — if not completely — plant-based diet. Those who follow a raw food plant-based diet eat only plant-based foods and do not eat animal foods, including dairy and eggs.

In general, raw food would constitute food that has not

been cooked over 115–120° F, so that the food would retain its natural enzymes.

There's a big debate in the raw food movement about how much raw food one should eat. So it's not surprising that I get this question often. People ask, "Is raw the way to go? What about 100% raw?" or "What should I be eating?"

Here's the simplest approach: in order to eliminate a lot of confusion around nutrition and science, the basis of your entire diet should be whole foods. Not super foods, not supplements, not anything else but whole foods — ripe, raw, uncooked, whole foods.

When it comes to what percentage should be raw, I recommend a *High Raw* approach. The concept of *High Raw* is hardly new. A *High Raw* food diet includes 75%–95% raw foods. The rest would include cooked, whole foods. Again, this might seem easy, but not if we get caught up in all of the confusion around nutrition. The biggest reason we might get confused by all of the conflicting information is if we forget to take a common sense approach.

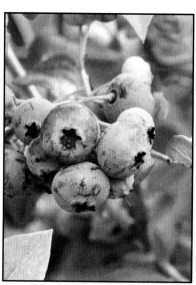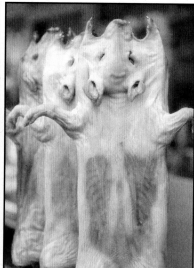

Here's an easy common sense experiment: Take a moment to look at the pictures on the previous page. Which would you rather eat?

Which of these foods looks more appetizing? You can make a common sense decision when you see the difference between the carnage of a cow vs. a nicely cut steak that's been pumped with carbon monoxide so it stays red longer. By the time you eat a steak, it looks nothing like where it came from. Yet the blueberries look exactly the same. All of the processing and manufacturing of our foods have simply removed us from nature and what is natural.

BACK TO NATURE & COMMON SENSE

If we were to go out into nature, we would pick our foods off a tree or perhaps pick it up off the ground, and we would eat it. We might have learned what is okay to eat from our ancestors, but if we didn't, we'd simply experiment. Experimenting might look like tasting something and seeing how we react. We'd be using our senses as a way to guide us to foods that work or don't work for each of us individually.

Today's modern diets are so full of processed foods that we have literally lost the connection to that process of experimenting. You may even feel like you've lost touch not only with what food is good, but also with what food is good for YOU personally.

Everyone worries about their health at times. So every time you feel like you're slipping off into worries like, "Should I be eating this or eating that?" With a *High Raw* approach, I invite you to reconnect to your senses and experiment. You will learn more about that in chapter 7. In the meantime, the easiest thing to embrace is this *High Raw* foundation: eat 75%–95% whole, ripe, raw foods.

> Worry and striving for perfection are two of the biggest pitfalls when it comes to sticking to your healthy diet.

The idea is to take this and use it as your foundation or a base that you can always come back to. Instead of worrying about what superfoods you should be eating, simply focus on your foundation and go from there.

I've found that the people who've been most successful with following a healthy diet embrace this foundation and what makes them really successful is they don't stress about it. Instead of worrying about perfection, they stick to a guidelines and principles. If you're worrying about being 100% raw or 100% anything, it can set you up on the wrong path. It is no longer fun...it's simply stressful. This is the point at which many people fail.

My goal is for you to create lasting success and one way to do that is to drop the worry and guilt—and enjoy your journey to good health. I'll give you an idea of how I've handled this in my own life. First of all, I don't worry about my diet because I always know I have a foundation. The foundation is to eat 75%–95% percent whole, ripe, raw foods. Now does that mean that I eat 75%–95% percent exactly and measure everything? Not at all! Instead, I may go for five days straight where I'll have everything raw and then maybe I'll have a cooked meal. Or perhaps I'll have two cooked meals and move on from there. When you follow the *High Raw* foundation, the beauty is that you don't need to be so specific and so scientific about it. What it DOES mean is that you have committed to a mindset to stick to a foundation for your healthy diet.

WHAT ABOUT THE SCIENCE OF RAW FOOD?

In terms of the *High Raw* lifestyle, I've done radio interviews with people and they ask me about the science of raw food.

I have to laugh about this because in a way, it's an absolutely ridiculous question.

Science and the *High Raw* lifestyle have an interesting relationship. Everyone talks about the science of raw food, and nutrition for that matter too. My question is this: is there really science around raw food? And more importantly, does there need to be? Do we need to break things down in order to understand that, for example, an apple picked from a tree is the most important thing for us? I don't think so.

When it comes to science and raw foods, you really only need to know one thing: You don't have to eat 100% raw foods to be healthy, but you do have to eat raw foods to be healthy.

Let's talk about some of the science around raw food:

- ENZYMES: Some people will argue that raw food is full of enzymes that make the food easier to digest and therefore, put less strain on your body.

- NUTRIENTS: Some people will argue that heat will destroy some of the vitamins and nutrients, like proteins. You will see plenty of studies showing that cooking can destroy vitamin C and B vitamins. Research has also shown that overcooking protein also affects its bio-availability by about 50%.[1]

> You don't have to eat 100% raw foods to be healthy, but you do have to eat raw foods to be healthy.

Cooking can also destroy tryptophan, the amino acid precursor to serotonin, known as the "feel good hormone" and melatonin, the "sleep hormone." Many people think that eating turkey makes them sleepy, but because tryptophan is largely destroyed by cooking, they are more likely sleepy due to overeating. A typical Thanksgiving meal, for example, includes massive amounts of carbohydrates, protein and fat, which overload your digestive system. It's no wonder people have to unbutton their pants before sitting down to watch the football game!

The science of raw food may tell us important things about nutrients and enzymes, but to be frank, I don't think we need to fill our heads with that information.

The reality is, before modern science even came along, we've had hundreds of thousands of years of nutritional symbiosis. That means that we have been in harmony with nature — and the food that nature has given us — for many, many years. Not only humans, but every other animal on the planet. A cat does not need to know if there's vitamin C in something or not. And do you think a cat needs to know all the different amino acids in the mouse that it finds out in the wild? It doesn't care. It just eats it.

From chapters 1 and 2, you already know that the foundation of science has some cracks and eventually, as it builds, it could crumble. As nutrition science continues to figure itself out, I think we're going to be left with what may feel like good old common sense: eat whole, raw, ripe, organic fruits, vegetables, nuts and seeds...the *High Raw* foundation. I like *High Raw* because it makes more sense for people. Again, not all science is bad — there is some science that is working — real scientific studies with human results...we just have to be alert and aware with any study we read.

One of the best studies that I've seen to date is *The China Study*, by T. Colin Campbell, Ph.D. The China Study is the largest epidemiological study ever, with surveys from 6,500 adults in more than 2,500 counties across China and Taiwan. Using hundreds of health and nutrition variables, *The China Study* draws links between diet and heart disease, cancer and diabetes.

The China Study began with an investigation into the unusually high incidence of liver cancer in children in the Philippines due to what they thought was high consumption of a mold toxin, called aflatoxins, in peanuts and corn. According to T. Colin Campbell, his findings in the Phillipines revealed something that flew in the face of science: "children who ate the highest protein diets were the most likely to get liver cancer!"[2] This discovery led to an in-depth scientific investigation into the affects nutrition on health.

The findings in The China Study were quite revealing about the link between nutrition and health:[3]

- People eating diets high in animal protein experienced more Western diseases, like cancer, heart attacks, hypertension and diabetes.

- People eating plant-based diets and plant-based protein were not suffering from Western diseases.

- Casein, which makes up 87% of cow's milk protein was the biggest promoter of cancer.

- Plant protein was the "safe" protein, which did not promote cancer.

- People who ate the most animal-based foods suffered most from chronic disease.

- People who ate the most plant-based foods were healthiest and did not tend to suffer from chronic disease.

- Healthy diet can reverse heart disease, diabetes and obesity and can benefit cancer, autoimmune disease, brain disorders, kidney health and bone health.

- A plant-based, whole foods diet has consistently shown to provide the most health benefits.

Is *The China Study* definitive? Like any study, we have to take it with a grain of salt. But is it the largest body of scientific evidence that we have? Yes. I think that's really important.

SO IS RAW REALLY THE WAY TO GO?

I'd like to eliminate all the raw food and vegan terminology and instead use the term, "plant-based" and *High Raw*.

Here are some of the basics of a High Raw plant-based diet:

- EAT WHOLE FOODS. Eat as close to nature as possible, choosing whole, unprocessed foods.

- EAT LOCALLY WHEN POSSIBLE. When possible, choose locally grown food. Here's the thing, because we as a people have been nomadic and moved all over this world, eating local is a good theory but it's not always realistic.

I interviewed Dr. Doug Graham about eating locally. A lifetime athlete, twenty-seven year raw fooder and author of *The 80/10/10 Diet*, Dr. Graham said that in reality, before houses with heat, we were nomadic people who migrated to the tropical climates in the winter. Now we heat our houses to tropical temperatures and live in cold climates. So if you live in Chicago in the winter, you'd hardly be able to eat locally. Do your best and enjoy local produce when you can.

- EAT ORGANIC. Organic foods are grown in mineral-rich soil and free of pesticides. They have more nutrients and less toxins, making it a much healthier option for your body.

- EAT A *HIGH RAW* DIET. Include 75%–95% raw, ripe fruit, vegetables, nuts and seeds in your diet.

Many people want to know where you'd get your protein if you eat a largely plant-based diet. I'm going to address this later in Chapters 4 and 5. For now, I'd like to point out that there are many sources of plant-based protein, such as: nuts, seeds, whole grains (like quinoa, for example, which has all 9 essential amino acids), sea vegetables (algae or seaweed), legumes, avocadoes and vegetables and even fruit. There are also many excellent plant-based, whole food protein supplements, like maca powder, brown rice protein, pea proteins, hemp seed and blue green algae.

GOOD FOR YOU, GOOD FOR THE PLANET

A *High Raw*, whole foods, plant-based diet is excellent for your health. And you know what else it's great for? The planet!

Think about it...the more whole foods you eat, the less packaging you'll use and the less trash you'll contribute. But that's not all. Eating a high animal-based protein diet has side effects for the planet and living things we share our planet with.

According to John Robbins, author of *Diet for a New America*, it takes approximately 2,500 gallons of water to produce a pound of meat.[4] Contrast that with the 25 gallons of water it takes to produce a pound of wheat and you can see the vast difference in resources that it takes to eat meat.

On top of that, John Robbins shares more reasons why a plant-based diet is better for the planet:

- For every quarter-pounder of meat consumes, an average of 55 square feet of tropical rainforest is destroyed.[5]

- 1,000 species become extinct each year because of tropical rainforest destruction for meat grazing and other uses.[6]

- It takes 50 times more fossil fuels to produce a meat-centered diet vs. a meat-free diet. Carbon dioxide from fossil fuels contributes to the greenhouse effect.[7]

A high animal-protein based diet is very wasteful. As you follow the *High Raw* principles, you may notice that you start to feel more connected to nature and the foods you eat. And as you educate yourself, which I cover in chapter 4, you'll start to realize how your eating habits effect more than just your health...they affect the planet's health as well. Once we all raise our awareness, we can literally save the planet. We will get to a point where environmental issues are no longer issues, just like your health...it all takes care of itself. That's the way it should be!

THE FIVE COMMON SENSE PRINCIPLES OF HIGH RAW

With the goal of keeping it simple and fun, *High Raw* is not about a complex set of numbers, calories or charts to memorize. Instead, I have created a common sense approach to creating your best health that is based on five principles.

Principles, also known as guiding principles, have long been used in high performing organizations to set a vision for success. You see, in any business, circumstances change and often, new situations arise for which a chart or formula no longer applies. Principles are about a way of thinking and taking action, regardless of the circumstances that arise. They are flexible so that you can meet the overlying goals, but allow for some wiggle room based on your unique situation.

THE FIVE PRINCIPLES OF HIGH RAW

In this chapter, I will give a brief overview of the Five Principles of *High Raw* and in chapters 5–9, I will provide detail for each chapter. Once you learn the Five Principles of *High Raw*, you may find that this whole "nutrition thing" feels a lot easier than you might have thought before. And certainly, you'll find that it can be much more fun than you might have imagined!

Here are the Five Principles of High Raw:

- **PRINCIPLE 1: EAT REAL FOOD & THINK LIKE A RAW FOODIST**
  First of all, this principle is about creating the mindset of a raw foodist. You don't have to be a raw foodist, but you want to create a mindset that helps you make decisions like someone who follows that type of diet. You'll get more tips on this in chapter 5. **In the meantime, here is what a raw foodist would be thinking when planning meals:**

  (1) 75%–95% whole, raw fruits, vegetables, nuts and seeds.

  (2) 0–20% cooked vegetables, steamed vegetables, cooked legumes and cooked grains.

  (3) 5% for FUN! Fun can mean more raw food or whatever else you want to put in there. Remember, you are creating the mindset of a raw foodist, so while in general, you'd be thinking about a raw food plant-based diet, for you, 5% fun might mean some animal protein. Fun might mean a dessert every once in a while. This is your time when you can play and enjoy yourself — and take a lighter approach to nutrition and health.

- **PRINCIPLE 2: MAKE YOUR HEALTH YOUR TOP PRIORITY**
  This is about figuring out what is most important to you when it comes to nutrition and health. Is your top priority being able to say, "I'm X% raw?" My guess is that it's more about feeling good, or something along those lines. What do you want to achieve? How do you want to feel? Find out what's important to you because what's

most important will be your biggest motivator in creating a lifestyle of healthy eating.

- **PRINCIPLE 3: KNOW YOUR BODY**
This is about really getting to know your own body, instead of relying solely on what everyone else tells you to do. There are several ways you can do this, which I'll cover in chapter 7. Once you know some key things about your body, you will feel even more empowered to make decisions about your health.

- **PRINCIPLE 4: EDUCATE YOURSELF**
This principle is about being your own health advocate by educating yourself about health and nutrition. With a few simple steps, you can become your own health expert so that you will not get caught up in second-guessing yourself every time you hear conflicting information from others.

- **PRINCIPLE 5: TAKE ACTION!**
Without this principle, nothing else will happen. Decide what you want to do and go out and do it. This is not about waiting until everything is perfect. It's about trusting what you know in this moment, deciding what you want to do and doing it. You'll learn more tips for taking action in chapter 9.

That's it — simple, isn't it? Health and nutrition does not have to be rocket science. We humans have been eating for thousands of years, before textbooks and scientific studies. But what our early ancestors had that we didn't is a deeper connection to the earth and to nature. As you learn and experiment with the *Five Principles of High Raw*, you too, will develop a deeper connection to nature. You may just find that you are guided toward what is best for you — the kind of guidance that comes from inside. Now what could be simpler than that?

It's fun to explore and learn — and there's a lot of information out there about nutrition and health. Over my years of research, I've read countless books and articles. And in the last eighteen months alone, I've interviewed 150 top experts. Each of these experts has worked with thousands of people and seen what works. So why make things complicated? The Five Principles of *High Raw* are the basis of everything I've learned, but simplified, so anyone can follow them.

CHAPTER 5

PRINCIPLE # 1: EAT REAL FOOD & THINK LIKE A RAW FOODIST

The first principle of *High Raw* is to eat real food and think like a *Raw Foodist*. Let's break this principle down for a moment.

You don't have to be a raw foodist, but you want to create a mindset that helps you make decisions like someone who follows that type of diet.

Using the *High Raw* ***approach, Principle #1 would look like this:***

(1) Eat 75%–95% whole, raw fruits, vegetables, nuts and seeds.

(2) Eat 0–20% cooked vegetables, steamed vegetables, cooked legumes and cooked grains.

(3) Use the remaining 5% for FUN! You decide what fun means to you. Whether it means more raw food, animal protein or dessert, this is your time to play and enjoy yourself.

But let's go below the surface for a moment because this principle is really about creating a mindset. The American Heritage Dictionary defines "mindset" as an inclination or habit. So you are essentially, setting up a habit or inclination to eat real food and think like a raw foodist.

As you know, once something is a habit, you tend to just do it automatically, without putting much thought into it. A perfect example of this is showering or brushing your teeth in the morning. Chances are you do this without much thought.

For your diet, it should be the same. Think about what this would look like for the first part of the principle: eating real food. Eating real food means eating as close to nature as possible: whole raw, ripe fruits, vegetables, nuts and seeds. Plants would make up most of your meals. As you eat closer to nature, you will find yourself drawn to foods that are organic and if available, locally grown. This may not happen overnight, but over time, as you create a habit of eating real food, you begin to feel your connection to the earth.

Right now, we are not talking about doing anything — we are talking about a way of thinking. As your thinking changes, it will influence your actions. That is why the first principle is about shifting your thinking...creating a habit of thought. We'll talk about translating that habit of thought into action in chapter 9.

HOW TO THINK LIKE A RAW FOODIST

So how does a raw foodist think when it comes to food choices? This isn't a complicated trivial pursuit question where you have to figure out the name of an obscure 19th century author. This is real simple stuff: a raw foodist would be planning meals around mostly fruits and vegetables.

To think like a raw foodist, consider these tips:

- BEFORE YOU START YOUR DAY OR PREPARE A MEAL, ask yourself, "What would a raw foodist eat right now? What would someone who eats fruits and vegetables eat right now?"

- GET A RAW FOOD RECIPE BOOK FOR IDEAS AND RECIPES. Getting a recipe book with pictures is a good place to start — because remember, you are creating a mindset. Even if you are not yet ready to take action, simply review the recipe book, look at the pictures and get ideas. Get to know what raw food plant-based meals look like. Start thinking about what your meals would look like if you were preparing these meals.

  One of my favorite recipe books for an exercise like this is: Nomi Shannon's *The Raw Gourmet*. *The Raw Gourmet* has a wide variety of raw food recipes for any occasion and plenty of full-color photographs to give you an idea of what raw food plant-based meals look like. And for live demonstrations, tune in to my blog, "The Renegade Health Show,"where my co-host and wife, Annmarie Gianni, and I show you how to make raw food meals from smoothies to burritos and more. On Wednesday nights, you can tune into www.RenegadeHealth.com for our weekly "In the Kitchen" episodes.

- NEXT TIME YOU GO SHOPPING, TAKE A WALK THROUGH THE PRODUCE AISLES AND LOOK AT THE VARIETY OF FRUITS AND VEGETABLES. If you aren't accustomed to eating a lot of fruits and vegetables, you may be surprised to see some produce you've never had before. Get a sense of what is there.

You might even consider going to your local health food store or farmer's market. Remember, you are creating a mindset — so focus on getting to know what's there and seeing what you may not have noticed before. Focus on raising your awareness about all of the options that are available to you. Have fun with it — maybe you'll even be adventurous and pick up something you've never had before.

IS THERE SOMETHING BETTER THAN THIS?

Let's face it, we live in a world that is full of fast food, convenience stores and vending machines. Most people are opening cans, bags or boxes to make a quick meal...or maybe picking something up from a drive through window. This is the typical mindset — fast and easy.

To make a shift in your diet and health, it will require moving from the prevailing mindset of processed foods that are literally everywhere, to venturing into health food stores or the far flung aisles of the grocery produce department.

In the introduction to this book, I shared my story. If you recall, my life changed dramatically after I awoke, hungover from a night of partying, and asked myself a simple question: "Is there something better than this?"

This is an important question to ask yourself as you create a mindset to eat real food and think like a raw foodist. That question will bring you a new awareness of the possibility that there might be something you can do to your meal — maybe to add one new thing into your meal that will give you a lot of benefits, that will help you get closer to your goal.

A MINDSET OF OPTIMAL HEALTH

If you think about it, your ultimate goal is not REALLY about being a raw foodist...more likely, your ultimate goal is optimal health. Sometimes, we can get so caught up in being healthy that we forget to have fun.

The first principle of *High Raw* is about creating a mindset for success — giving you a guideline to have the highest percentage of your meals as whole, raw, ripe fruits, vegetables, nuts and seeds. How you work the percentages is up to you, but remember to include 5% fun!

Where could you go wrong? Where I've seen people go

wrong is when they chase perfection. If you're chasing something like 100% raw food or a 100% strict diet — 100% of anything leaves very little wiggle room to allow yourself to address what you need in any given moment. The mindset it often creates is "all or nothing," which can ultimately sabotage your success.

Being able to say, "I'm 100% raw" or "I have six pack abs" does not really mean much if you aren't feeling your best AND enjoying the journey. So what would it look like if you shifted your focus to feeling your best? This means feeling your best emotionally and physically. How would it change your actions if you were simply focusing on creating optimal health?

The true reward is how you feel when you're ON the journey. Now if your goal is to feel your best and being 100% raw is doing that for you, then go for it! The key here is to switch your focus on labeling what you are doing and focus on how you feel.

While health is a serious topic, we don't have to be so serious about it. Give yourself permission to trust that you are creating a mindset of healthy habits and allow yourself to enjoy the journey!

WHERE COULD YOU GO WRONG?

Where I've seen people go wrong is when they chase perfection. If you're chasing something like 100% raw food or a 100% strict diet — 100% of anything leaves very little wiggle room to allow yourself to address what you need in any given moment. The mindset it often creates is "all or nothing," which can ultimately sabotage your success.

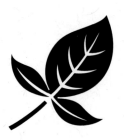

CHAPTER 6

PRINCIPLE #2: MAKE YOUR HEALTH YOUR TOP PRIORITY

In Stephen Covey's bestseller, The 7 Habits of Highly Effective People, the third habit is "put first things first." Covey and many other success experts say that given all of the things we have on our "to do" lists, the only things that will really get done are those that we prioritize.

Principle #2 is about making your health your top priority. Think about something that's really important to you. If you are a person who exercises regularly, you have surely decided at some point that fitness is important — so you fit it into your day, even if you have a busy schedule (and who doesn't these days?). If you are a parent and your child is sick, you would move aside your work schedule to take care of your child. That's because your kids are a priority. It doesn't mean your work goes away that day, but you find a way to work it out.

When something is important to you, you are motivated to make it happen in spite of all of the other things competing for your time. When something is important to you, you will say no to whatever tries to get in the way.

In chapter 5, we talked about creating a mindset for

optimal health. So what would it look like if this were your top priority? Remember what you read in chapter 5 — optimal health is not about labeling yourself. It's not about saying, "I'm X% raw" or putting a plaque on your wall that says, "I'm a raw foodist." None of this really matters — because what matters most is how you feel. If it's your top priority to feel great — to have optimal health, it will be important to you. You will make time for it each day.

So take a moment and ask yourself some questions:

- How do I feel?
- Am I feeling my best emotionally and physically?
- What would it be like to feel my best?
- How important is it to feel my best?
- What are my priorities right now?
- If I want to feel my best, am I willing to make it my top priority?
- If optimal health were my top priority, what would I be doing differently?

What we all seem to want is to feel our best, don't we? If you can answer, "yes, I feel my best," then keep doing whatever it is you are doing. You'll know you're on the right track with anything if you feel your best.

IF YOU WANT SOMETHING, YOU'LL MAKE IT HAPPEN

The reality of it is if you want something, you can make it happen. Nothing will get in the way. If you don't have the money, you'll find a way to make the money. If you don't have the skills, you'll find a way to get the skills. If you don't know the right people, you'll find a way to meet them. When you want something badly enough, you'll do whatever it takes, right?

Dan Kennedy, marketing expert and author of seven business books, really put the power of priorities into perspective for me when he said that if you drive through a very depressed neighborhood in a big city, there are two things that you will notice: even if all the housing is section eight (subsidized housing for low income families), a good portion of them have satellite dishes and nice cars. Not even money will get in the way, if they have decided these things are their priorities.

MOVING BEYOND EXCUSES AND CREATING PRIORITIES:

- If you want to feel your best, what is getting in the way? Time? Money? Knowledge? Motivation? Fear of failure? Fear or success? _____ (fill in the blank)?
- What would happen if those things were not in the way?

If any of these things get in the way of your health, then the real issue is one of priorities. Because if your health were your top priority, you'd go after it, regardless of what might get in the way.

If we haven't prioritized something, we can use a lot of excuses as to why we aren't doing it. Zig Ziglar, speaker and author of twenty-seven books on personal growth, leadership, sales, faith, family and success, calls this "stinking thinking." And according to Zig Ziglar, this can cause a hardening of attitudes. Basically, you stop seeing the opportunities and focus on the excuses. But if you make something a priority, you will not let excuses get in the way.

If you are ready to make your health your top priority, you CAN get there — I know you can! No one said that change is easy — and it's certainly not about being perfect all the time — or doing the right thing all the time. The idea is to decide what's important and make that your priority. Things might get in the way...there might be issues of money, time, knowledge and on some days, maybe even motivation. But when you want it enough, you'll work through those to make it happen anyway. And the good news is, that I will cover tips for each of these in chapters 10 and 11 — to set you up for success.

I've had my share of challenges along the way to great health and believe me, if I can do it, so can you! Chapters 10 –13 are chock full of tips that I've learned over the years to keep you focused on your priorities, no matter what!

CHAPTER 7

PRINCIPLE #3: KNOW YOUR BODY

Principle #3 is about knowing your body — what's happening in your body and what works for you personally. This is key because if you don't know your body, you can too easily second guess yourself every time you hear another person's opinion.

Imagine going back in time, when there was no nutrition science...no experts to tell you what you should eat. Keep in mind that back then, just under 200 years ago, you wouldn't have the proliferation of processed foods and fast food. Sugar was a rare treat. Back then, you would more likely be eating whole foods that were organic and local. You might even be growing your own food. In other words, you'd be closer to nature.

Instead of looking up the science of the foods you ate, you'd listen to your body — because that's about all you could do. Doctors were not even as accessible as they are today. Today, we are lucky to have the acute care that Western medicine provides. But back then, without the access you have today, you might be a little more aware of how the foods you ate affected you.

The signs and symptoms that foods might not agree with you are really not all that mysterious, if you pay attention to them.

Here are some examples:

- **Skin:** rash, itching, acne, hives, eczema, psoriasis
- **Respiratory:** difficulty breathing, coughing
- **Digestive:** indigestion, abdominal pain, constipation, diarrhea
- **Mouth:** tongue (color, coating) and changes in teeth like cavities, discoloration, sensitivity to hot and cold
- **Eyes:** look for color and irritations — red, itchy, watering.
- **Urinary:** notice deviations from the typical yellow color, like red, pink, orange, green, dark brown, murky or cloudy. For example, if your urine is dark you could be dehydrated or you could have an issue with your liver. Supplements, food and medication may affect the color of your urine.
- **Energy:** fatigue, restlessness, sleep patterns
- **Emotions:** depression, anxiety, stress, panic

Your body is constantly giving you signals about what foods and drinks are best for you. You will also get physical and emotional symptoms if you are under too much stress or living a lifestyle that does not support your happiness. So Principle #3 — Know Your Body, is about paying attention to your body. Whether you know it or not, you have intuition. While we are not equipped like cars, with a dashboard that tells about temperature, fuel, speed or engine issues, we do have these incredible physical and emotional signals to tell us how we're doing.

Think of your body's signals like a car's dashboard. Start checking in by tuning in to how you feel. This is a great way to develop your intuition and get a better sense of how food and your lifestyle are affecting your health.

Here's how:

- Several times per day, check in and see how you feel physically and emotionally. How's your energy? Are you feeling good? Are you experiencing any symptoms?

- Check in before meals and directly after meals.

- Check in again a couple hours after meals.

- Write down what you learn, so you can keep track.

- If you do experience symptoms, write them down. Then ask yourself: is there something I ate or something I'm doing that might contribute to this? For example, you might experience symptoms after breakfast, but you also felt stressed as you rushed to work. It will be important to identify if it was the stress in rushing to work or the food that created those symptoms.

The truth is, most of us have become so disconnected from our bodies that when symptoms arise, they seem very mysterious. We wonder what is wrong or maybe, pop a pill to feel better. The more you tune into your body, the more you will be able to identify links between your food, lifestyle and symptoms — and then you can make adjustments to feel better. If you continue to practice this over time, you will find that you are simply drawn to what works for you because you know your body so well.

DEVELOPING YOUR INTUITION — THE TWO-WEEK EXPERIMENT APPROACH

As you get used to sensing what is happening in your body, you can take it a step further with an approach that has been very successful for me: the two-week experiment.

Let's say for example, that you love pizza and you're not sure if it's causing symptoms. Stop eating it for two weeks and then, after the two weeks, introduce a small amount of pizza back into your diet and see how you feel:

- Do you get a stomachache?

- Do you get acne?

- Do you get diarrhea?

The two-week experiment is the way that I check in with my body periodically, to see how certain foods are affecting my body. I do this in two ways:

(1) If I start noticing symptoms, I'll stop eating a certain food for two weeks to see if the symptoms subside. If they do, I'll know which food was causing those symptoms. The key is to stop just one food at a time, so you'll know if that particular food is linked to the symptoms.

(2) If I want to introduce a certain food I haven't had in awhile, that my body is not used to, I'll take a small amount and see how I feel for two weeks. The key here is that I choose one type of food during the experiment and I only have a small amount. (I've done this experiment with goat cheese as well as processed sugar to confirm that the latter definitely does not work with me!)

Doing two-week experiments has been very instructive for me because I've learned which foods wreak havoc with my body and as you can imagine, it's not something I want to repeat too often!

In your experiment with pizza, notice how your body feels when you don't eat pizza and then when you introduce it again. Pay attention to changes in your body, your energy and your moods. This is an incredible way to learn your boundaries — which foods are most supportive of feeling your best.

I did my first two-week experiment after a seminar with Tony Robbins in Secaucus, New Jersey. A great motivational speaker, Tony asked the question, "What if you eliminated dairy for two weeks? Would you feel better?" Caught up in the excitement, I went right home and tried it for myself. I didn't know what to expect, but what I learned was amazing. At the time, I had some razor burn under my chin — kind of like whiteheads — that bled and got irritated when I shaved. It was pretty gross and I had no idea where it was coming from. I figured, maybe it was a little acne and that it was probably just normal.

After eliminating dairy for two weeks, the razor burn went away! I was amazed. After the two weeks, I was with my friends and I decided it was time to celebrate with some pizza. I had six slices — I admit, I love to eat! Well, what happened after that was very instructive. My stomach hurt so much that I'm not sure it will ever forgive me for that transgression. On top of that, the razor burn returned. You can imagine that I was pretty motivated to eliminate dairy entirely and I did. A year later, I experimented again with the same symptoms of stomach upset and razor burn, so today, dairy is not in my diet.

Doing two-week experiments is also how I found out that I don't do well with processed sugar. I'm actually okay with the naturally occurring sugar in fruit, but processed sugar makes me feel wired and hyper. If you currently eat sugar, I invite you to do your own two-week experiment with sugar and see how you feel. It's probably one of the easiest experiments to track the difference in how you feel.

USING THE SCIENTIFIC PROCESS FOR YOURSELF

As you are learning to sense what is happening in your body, there are also some really great scientific tests that can help establish a baseline for how your body is doing. Using a combination of tuning into your body and scientific testing can go hand in hand for allowing you to target solutions for your health goals.

First, it's important to know a few things about the testing options:

- **NOT ALL TESTS ARE ACCURATE.** For example, the most common test for Lyme disease is an antibody test called the Enzyme Linked Immune Sera Assay test (ELISA). An ELISA test study by Lori Bakken showed that while labs often claim 99% accuracy, ELISA is only 50% accurate.[1]

    In a case like Lyme Disease, symptoms may be a better indicator than the ELISA. According to the Centers for Disease Control and Prevention (CDC), "The majority of patients with Lyme disease develop symptoms like: erythema migrans (EM), fever, malaise, fatigue, headache, myalgia, or arthralgia. Other manifestations of infection can include arthritis, carditis, and neurologic deficits."[2]

- **TESTS ARE VALUABLE FOR GIVING YOU A BASELINE.** In this chapter, I am going to cover some very valuable tests and the thing to keep in mind is that they will give you a baseline. While it's true that not all tests are accurate, they give you a place to start, an indicator. Let's say you are experiencing mood issues and you get a test where your levels of vitamin B6 are low. You and your health care practitioner decide to use supplements and your diet to boost your vitamin B6 levels. When you go back and get tested again, you can see if the dietary and supplement strategy actually helped to boost your levels of vitamin B6. Of course, you will also be looking for physical and emotional symptoms, but you'll get validation from your testing. In other words, even if the number itself is not accurate, you'll be able to see if the numbers go up or down.

Another reason that tests can be helpful in establishing a baseline is the standard reference range. The reference range tells you if you are in the range of what is considered normal for your age, gender or other categories. Small changes within the reference range may be no cause for concern in most cases, but they can still give you important information. For example, if your thyroid tests showed within the reference range, and two years later you experienced symptoms of low thyroid, you could be tested again. In your second test, if your thyroid results were lower, you'd understand why you were experiencing symptoms — even if the results were still within the normal reference range. Without the baseline test, your doctor would just say, "your results are normal" and you'd wonder what was going on. Since you have the baseline test, you and your doctor can see that for you personally, there has been a change.

If you have a baseline test with results in the normal range and then subsequent tests show results outside the reference range, you'd really want to look into what's happening with your health care practitioner. So you can see how valuable baseline testing is — it is a way for you to gain insight into what's happening in your body.

- TESTS CAN HELP YOU WITH CHOOSING A HEALTH PROTOCOL. One of the dangers I see is when people go online to search for symptoms they are experiencing and then choose a protocol based on what they find online. While I am an advocate of people taking responsibility for their health, I am not an advocate of jumping into a protocol without any validation about the root cause of symptoms.

For example, I was reading one of the Master Cleanse websites that outlined several different benefits of the Master Cleanse. The Master Cleanse is a popular detoxification program that includes a protocol of drinking a lemonade made of lemons, cayenne pepper, maple syrup and sea salt. This website claimed that one of the symptoms of detoxification is "hot stools" and that it meant toxins were being removed from your body. What's so interesting about claims like this is that they spread misinformation like wildfire. Anyone eating foods with hot spices, like cayenne pepper can experience hot stools. As a football fan who used to consume a lot of hot wings, I could have told you that!

When it comes to natural health, there are plenty of great products, websites and information. However, there is also a lot of misinformation that leads to following protocols that may end up confusing you more than helping you. Testing can help in determining what protocol is right for your unique needs.

OPTIONS FOR TESTING

Here are some tests are really helpful in getting to know your body:

- COMPLETE BLOOD PROFILE. Also called a Complete Blood Count (CBC), this is a test I highly recommend. The complete blood profile measures the concentration of white blood cells, red blood cells, and platelets in your blood. This test is often used to identify the general state of your health, find an infection, identify whether symptoms are related to certain diseases, provide indicators of hydration or dehydration or reactions to inflammation.

You can have a complete blood profile done by a health professional, like a doctor (MD), naturopath or nutritionist. The test itself is simple: your blood is drawn and your results will be sent to your health practitioner, who will help you interpret the results. If you see any irregularities then you know that you may need to address something specifically. If you don't that doesn't necessarily mean you don't have any problems or any challenges, but it's one baseline that you can use.

I recommend that you get a complete blood profile once a year. One company that does complete blood profile tests in the United States is Lab Corp, which you can find online at www.labcorp.com.

- VITAMIN AND MINERAL LEVELS. A nutritional evaluation can identify whether you have vitamin, mineral and essential co-factor imbalances. It can be very valuable to know if you have mineral deficiencies, like sodium, potassium, magnesium, iron, calcium, and phosphate, for example. Mineral deficiencies can lead to several symptoms, chief among them is fatigue or low energy. Direct Labs is one lab in the United States that does vitamin and mineral testing.

Two important vitamin level tests for those following a plant-based or raw food diet (because these vitamins are mainly found in animal products like meat, fish and dairy) are:

(1) **Vitamin B12.** It is common for vegetarians and raw foodists to have low B12 levels, but anyone can be low in B12. I will cover the importance of B12, why you could be deficient and signs of B12 deficiency in chapter 15. Getting tested can help you identify if you are low in vitamin B12, which

has important functions for your mood, energy levels and nervous system.

While there are several tests for vitamin B12 deficiency, the most sensitive is Methylmalonic Acid (MMA). The MMA is a non-invasive urine test. Sally M. Pacholok, R.N. and Jeffrey J. Stuart, D.O., authors of the book, *Could it Be B12?: An Epidemic of Misdiagnosis* recommend *Norman Clinical Laboratory* (www.b12.com) for getting MMA testing by mail.

Choose the Most Accurate test for B12 Deficiency:[3]

1. Serum B12: this measures the B12 in your blood serum and can give false negative or false positive results. There are also discrepancies in what is considered low B12 levels.

2. Serum MMA: This measures the amount of methylmalonic acid (MMA) in your blood serum and can result in false positives or false negatives.

3. Urinary MMA: This is the most accurate of the tests for B12 because MMA is 40 times more concentrated in your urine than in your blood. This measures the amount of methylmalonic acid in your urine and the test does not result in false negatives or false positives.

(2) **Vitamin D.** Vitamin D deficiency is more common than you think. I will cover more about vitamin D deficiency, including symptoms, in chapter 15. Your health practitioner can order this test for you. Direct Labs (www.directlabs.com) is one lab in the United States that does vitamin D testing.

- **C-Reactive Protein.** Also known as CRP, the c-reactive protein test is used to diagnose signs of inflammation that play a role in cardiovascular disease, stroke, some forms of arthritis, lupus, inflammatory bowel disease, autoimmune disease and pelvic inflammatory disease. A CRP is a simple blood test that people sometimes get when they are getting their cholesterol tested. Direct Labs does CRP testing.

- **Heavy Metals.** Heavy metal toxicity can cause a variety of symptoms, like digestive pain, nausea, headaches, sweating and candida. A good test for heavy metals is the hair test because it is the most accurate. Doctor's Data, Inc. is a lab that does hair testing for heavy metals.

The complete blood profile has been beneficial in my own health by helping me address low minerals. For candida (a systemic yeast infection), the tests that helped me were the IgA, IgG and the IgM assay, which test for antibodies to Candida albicans.. If I hadn't had scientific tests to back up the root cause of the symptoms I was experiencing, I'd still be struggling today. With scientific testing, I have been able to work through these symptoms in a much more targeted (and much easier!) way.

The more scientific information that you can gather about your health, the more you'll know your body. The more that you know your body, the more you'll be able to tweak and adjust. For instance, if you took a complete blood profile every year for ten years, you could look at every year and see where you're fluctuating.

Checking your cholesterol levels is a good example. If you noticed your cholesterol continued to rise, you could start addressing it right away — before there were any health issues, like a heart attack.

Fifty percent of men and 64 percent of women who died suddenly of coronary heart disease had no previous symptoms of this disease.[3] Testing can be a great asset in disease prevention, in addition to helping you stay on track with your health. Whether you have health insurance or not, I like to think of testing as a kind of "health insurance" because it can help prevent future health issues that could otherwise go unnoticed.

If you don't have a practitioner you can go to a company called Direct Labs (www.directlabs.com) and you can get the tests mailed directly to you. Direct Labs will send you to a local lab, like Lab Corp, where they will take your blood, urine or whatever is being tested. Once the analysis is complete, you will receive the results by mail.

Once you are armed with the test results, going online and researching what the information means is a much better process than surfing the web without really knowing what is going on. The results aren't that difficult to read, but it can be helpful to have a health practitioner review and interpret them with you.

WHY WORK WITH A HEALTH PRACTITIONER?

I prefer working with a health practitioner. I like to think of a health practitioner as any professional I'd go to for advice. If I were building a business, I might hire a consultant with expertise in marketing, business strategy or accounting. If I were an athlete, I might hire a coach to motivate and support me in improving my performance. A student might hire a tutor to improve performance on tests. When it comes to your health, having an expert — a coach, a health practitioner — can be a tremendous asset in helping you achieve your goals. An expert can greatly shortcut the learning curve and make your journey much easier. They've seen things thousands of times and may be able to interpret tests or symptoms in ways you'd never have been able to imagine on your own.

People who work with experts — health practitioners, coaches or mentors, are able to realize improvements faster. Think of the most successful people you know. Chances are, they have all been coached or mentored in some way. They have all worked with experts who help them bring out their best. Michael Phelps, who won 14 career Olymic gold metals in swimming worked with many of the best coaches. The same is true for Tiger Woods. And in business, billionaire Richard Branson, who created the Virgin brand of over 360 companies, had mentors along the way to his success.

Success comes from learning from other people's experiences. When you reach out to people, whether in person, over the phone or even online, you may find that achieving your goals is easier and much more fun.

MANAGING MONEY — CAN YOU AFFORD TO DO TESTING?

If your medical doctor orders tests for you, they may be covered by your health care insurance (or at least a percentage of the cost). However, I know that not everyone has health insurance. I firmly believe that the value of these tests far outweigh the cost and yet, I am also aware that everyone has a different perspective about money. I have often been asked, "Can I afford these tests?" But the real question is, when it comes to your health, can you afford not to?

When you make your health your top priority (*High Raw* Principle #2), you may find that you are able to come up with the money you need. Just remember, you don't need to do all of these tests at once. Go at the pace that works for you. I will address more about money and health in chapter 13.

We've all heard that patience is a virtue and yet, it is often difficult to be patient when you've started working toward your goals. It's actually really easy to get caught up in wanting to hurry things along, cut to the chase, be done with it already.

When it comes to your health, it's important to give your body time to heal. Since everyone is different, the amount of time it takes you may be very different from the amount of time it takes someone else. Once you get your test results and start working on your health protocol, I recommend listening to your body and taking it slowly. Part of enjoying the journey is allowing yourself to heal at the pace that's right for your body.

Let's say you get your test results and you begin a protocol. After three days, are you already looking for results? If you don't see results immediately, are you on to the next thing? The danger here is that you will jump around so much that your body can't catch up and heal at its own pace. You also put yourself and your body through a lot of unnecessary stress.

Think about the two-week experiment approach. Commit to giving yourself at least two weeks to see if something is going to work before moving on to the next thing. If you have a serious illness or find that you are feeling really confused, I recommend working with a health practitioner. In situations like this, working with an expert can support you in setting a time frame that works for your healing protocol.

Most importantly, remember not to take your health too seriously. Instead, trust that you have committed to the *High Raw* Principle #2 and your health is your top priority. Once you trust this, you can focus on taking on a curious, explorative, lighthearted mindset. As you track your results, consider writing in a journal about what you're learning and how you are feeling. If some symptoms are going away, celebrate that! We sometimes forget to celebrate milestones on the way to the end game.

Here's what I did in order to address Lyme disease and candida:

- CANDIDA. I reviewed all of the natural healing protocols for candida, selected four of them and took the two-week experiment approach for each. Some of the protocols were better than others, but the good news is that I stuck with it and eliminated candida.

- LYME DISEASE. I took the same two-week experiment approach and in this case, I worked with four health coaches. Two of the coaches I worked with alone had over 60 years of experience in helping thousands of clients, so you can imagine I trusted what they had to say! In the end, I chose a natural treatment, combined with antibiotics.

Overall, I am grateful that candida and Lyme disease were part of my journey because not only did I learn a lot about what works for me, I also felt empowered to take charge of my health.

The more you get to know your body, the more you will trust the signals of your body. And as you trust your body, it may be easier to be patient and allow your results to unfold at your body's pace. Scientific testing and health experts can help guide you along the journey. And if you can express gratitude for what you are learning along the way — for getting to know yourself better and for accomplishing your health goals, you may find that this whole journey to "being healthy" feels a lot easier.

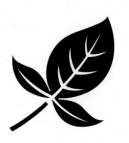

CHAPTER 8

PRINCIPLE #4: EDUCATE YOURSELF

Principle #4 is about educating yourself. Why is this so important? After reading chapters 1 and 2, it's pretty clear that there is a lot of confusing and conflicting information out there about health and nutrition. And think about it... you are probably surrounded by people who will be happy to give you their opinions about what is or is not healthy.

How many times have you been at the dinner table with your family and suddenly nutrition came up? What happens if one of your family members starts arguing exactly the opposite of a point you were making? Believe me, I've been there! And I can guarantee that if you want to avoid second-guessing yourself and constantly being swayed by opposing opinions, it's critical to be your own health expert.

Chances are, your family members haven't read all that much about nutrition. Perhaps they are getting their information from TV or newspaper headlines from press releases! You and I know how faulty these sources can be. The truth is, most of the people you encounter each day don't read much about nutrition. If you're not sure about this, do your own experiment: ask them, "How many books on nutrition have you read in the past five years?" Don't be surprised if the answer is none or perhaps, one.

For most people, the only education they've had on health and nutrition was sixth grade health class. Perhaps they've seen the food pyramid and this is what they've committed to memory. Well, after reading chapter 2, you know how much the lobbyists have influenced even the food pyramid. So what the average person knows about health has been based on a lot of the "swaying" of science and the media that we've already covered.

To be honest, I would rather talk about politics AND religion at the dinner table than I would about nutrition. Because most of the time, you end up talking to someone who only knows what the media has convincingly sold them. If you haven't educated yourself about health and nutrition, it may be too easy to be convinced during conversations like these.

The key to Principle #4 is that your own education is your responsibility. You can't let anyone else take the responsibility to educate you. So how do you go about educating yourself when there is so much confusing information out there? First of all, the more you read and learn, the more you will gain insight into which sources are reputable. Additionally, you will learn with sources resonate with YOU. That's really important too. And finally, as you put the Five Principles of *High Raw* into action, especially Principle #3: Know Your Body, you will start to understand what works for you specifically.

Here are some tips for educating yourself in health and nutrition:

- SCHEDULE TIME TO LEARN. Plan your learning by putting it on your calendar. Remember Principle #2 — Prioritize Your Health. When you know your health is important to you, you'll make time for it. Scheduling time in your daily planner will keep you on track with your learning.

- **FIND MENTORS.** Seek out some key experts who you trust. Choose mentors who have years of expertise and can help you learn faster. Listen to multiple people. I always tell people not to just listen to me or to one person — but to go out there and talk to many people. You'll gain a lot of insights from hearing different points of view or even the same information presented in different ways.

- **ASK YOUR MENTORS FOR READING SUGGESTIONS.** A great way to find good sources of nutrition and health information is to ask your mentors or other experts for suggestions. You can even review the bibliography of their books or sources of articles they have written.

- **BE CURIOUS.** Be like a sponge and soak up the information you find. Keep an open mind, but take everything with a grain of salt. Remember that everyone is different and trust what works for you specifically.

- **BE COMFORTABLE WITH CONFUSION.** When you go out there and educate yourself, you will start to see all of the conflicting information. You may also learn new things that seem really confusing. That's okay! Every time you learn something new, it feels confusing at first — you are moving out of your comfort zone and stretching yourself. Be comfortable with confusion and trust that as you continue learning, you will put the pieces in place and learn to trust what you know.

- **START YOUR OWN HEALTH JOURNAL.** Take notes on key points that you learn from books, events and conversations with other health experts. Keeping a health journal allows you to have one place with all of the information you are learning.

- **START A HEALTH "BOOK CLUB".** A lot of people belong to book clubs. What if you started a book club to discuss what you learned about health? This could help motivate you to learn a lot and give you others to discuss your learnings with. Remember that not all people will agree with everything they read. This is good and will provide healthy discussion. As you master the *Five Principles of High Raw*, you'll be able to determine what you resonate with.

- **BE CREATIVE.** Use tools to help you. I like to use visuals. If you are a visual learner, draw pictures or flow charts to show relationships of what you are learning. Make charts or tables to categorize the information so you can see the basics at a glance.

EVEN THE EXPERTS DISAGREE

The more you educate yourself about health and nutrition, the more you will see that even health experts you like will disagree on certain points. Whether it's about how much fruit to eat, whether to consume grains or how to combine certain foods, there will be plenty of experts who teach the exact opposite of one another.

When listening to a talk between Joel Fuhrman, author of *Eat for Health* and *Eat to Live*, and John McDougall, author of *The McDougall Program for Maximum Weight Loss* and *Dr. McDougall's Digestive Tune-Up*, they were arguing about the amount of grains to include in one's diet. It's not uncommon that two advocates of the plant-based diet could agree on 99.9% of everything, but still disagree on one small point.

This is going to happen, so instead of getting frustrated, simply accept that there will be disagreement. I'd much rather help people change their lives than argue about small points that make nutrition too complicated.

As you master the Five Principles of *High Raw*, you will no longer get caught up in all of the arguments because you'll know what works for you. And of course, when you take a light-hearted approach to nutrition, you'll be too busy having fun to get caught up in arguments!

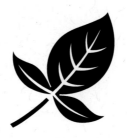

CHAPTER 9

PRINCIPLE #5: TAKE ACTION!

You see, in life, lots of people know what to do, but few people actually do what they know. Knowing is not enough! You must take action.
—ANTHONY ROBBINS

Principle #5 is perhaps the most important principle of all: Take Action! Once you have mastered the first four principles of *High Raw*, the fifth principle is how you make them work for you. It's important to keep in mind that you do not need to have all your ducks in a row before you take action. This is not about perfection! This is about getting started by taking one small step at a time. If you wait until you know everything there is to know, you may never get started at all.

The vast majority of successful people take a ready, fire, aim approach to life. They get just enough information, create a plan and get out there and do it. Most of the time, they don't have all the information they need, but they gather it along the way. And they make adjustments along the way. They may even make some mistakes along the way, but they learn from their mistakes and keep progressing. If you are waiting to get your Ph.D. in nutrition before you take any action or make a change, you could be waiting a very long time.

Action is important because it is the catalyst to your success. How long have you been thinking about your health, but not taking action? Maybe you are feeling like I did all those years ago when I lived in that basement in Brooklyn... I knew there was something wrong and I even knew what I needed to do. But I didn't take action and to be honest, I was simply afraid to make a change in any direction. I wondered what would happen if I stopped drinking or if I moved home. The thing is, I couldn't have known how much better it would be unless I actually did something! Turns out, when I moved home, the worst thing that happened was my mother would not let me put my clothes in the dresser. She wanted me to recognize that this was temporary. And when I stopped drinking, I managed to get a clear head and take steps toward creating a rewarding business.

Today, I look back and wonder what would have happened if I stayed stuck in inaction. Action brings opportunity — and certainly, it has its own set of challenges. The difference is that when you are taking action, you are in the driver's seat. There is an empowerment that comes with moving toward your goals.

I've seen this happen again and again with my clients in my personal training and health coaching business. My wife, Annmarie, and I approach our clients by first identifying their goals. In personal training, it's usually about weight loss or building muscle. Once their goals are defined, we start talking to them about the action steps they can take to get there, including fitness, health and nutrition. What we found over the years is that our clients who were consistently successful, got results simply because they took action. We gave them guidance, tools and action steps — but their success hinged on creating a habit of action.

The habit of action has nothing to do with a specific food they ate or a specific exercise they did.

Instead, the habit of action has to do with:

- IDENTIFYING THE CHANGE YOU WANT TO MAKE. You don't have to have the answers, you simply have to have the right questions (see below for more on this).

- DECIDING WHAT STEPS YOU WANT TO TAKE. Make sure you are not getting caught up in "analysis paralysis" where you feel you have to have 100% of the answers before you get started. Pick something you can take action on immediately.

- PUTTING A SYSTEM IN PLACE TO FOLLOW THROUGH WITH THOSE STEPS. Hold yourself accountable for taking action. Put it on your calendar and check in with yourself. Eventually, as you create new habits, you will do them automatically.

- MAKING ADJUSTMENTS AS NEEDED. As you take action, you will learn what does or does not work for you.

- BEING CONSISTENT. When you commit to taking action, you consistently follow the steps you decided to take, at least long enough to see if they work for you. Giving yourself time to stick with your plans allows you to see if they will work for you. The general guideline for creating a new habit is to be consistent for 21 days.

START WITH THE RIGHT QUESTIONS

What sets successful people apart is not that they have all the answers...it's that they ask themselves the right questions.

Here are some examples of questions I always ask myself:
- "What can I do tomorrow that will help me reach my goals?"
- "How can I improve my health?"
- "What can I do to get healthier right now?"
- "Who can help me improve my health?"

- "What can I do to get the best water possible?"
- "How can I help more people today?"
- "What's the best way to get the best results?"
- "What's the fastest way to feel better?"

What do you notice about these questions? First of all, the fact that I am asking them means I am starting, not from a place of having the answers, but from the place of having the questions. You don't need to have all the answers to make changes in your life!

Second, in some cases, I am asking who can help me. Remember, you don't have to take action completely on your own. Just like I mentioned in chapter 8, working with a mentor, coach or expert can really help – because you can take action a lot faster when you are being guided by someone who's been there. If you wait until you have 100% certainty or all the answers, you will miss out on the adventure of getting out there and seeing what will happen by taking just one step toward your goal.

To make changes in your life, all you need to have are the questions. If you can ask yourself these questions, guess what's going to happen? You're going to get amazing answers.

However, beware of asking yourself the kind of questions that keep you stuck. Here are some examples of questions that keep you stuck:
- "Why do I feel so lazy?"
- "What's wrong with me?"
- "Why can't I lose weight?"
- "Why am I so unhealthy?"
- "Why can he do it, but I can't?"

- "Why does it have to be so hard?"
- "Why am I so stressed out?"

Have you ever asked yourself questions like these? We all have...and as you think about these questions, what happens? The answers you give yourself are likely to be negative. You are likely to start dumping on yourself for all of the reasons you CAN'T make a change.

These are questions that keep you stuck because they generate fear and doubt. You are now focused on the worst parts of yourself, rather than the best. Take a look again at the first set of questions and notice how different they are. Would you rather ask yourself, "Why do I feel so lazy?" or "What can I do tomorrow that will help me reach my goals?" Which question inspires you to take action?

Let's use an example. Think about the last time you were feeling down about yourself. Maybe you were watching TV or just in the car and you thought about something that made your self-esteem drop. Chances are you asked yourself a question at that moment... and it probably was something like, "Why does this always happen to me?" or something similar.

A question like that is not a great question because the answer will support your low self esteem. So your answers could be... "because, I'm lazy," or "because, I'm always procrastinating," etc.

A good question to reverse that negativity and change your pattern would be "How can I raise my self esteem today?"

Imagine the answers that you could come up with now.

EXPECTING RESULTS

Let's face it, most of us want results immediately, don't we? The thing is, when you are making changes in your life, you don't always get immediate results. Sometimes, it can feel like you take two steps forward and one step back. The reality is, results come over time and they require steady, consistent action. While you may notice some immediate results, you will more likely experience results over time. If you stick with it and trust the goals that you set for yourself, you will enjoy the journey much more than if you place expectations on when you should see results.

When it comes to your health, the old fable of the tortoise and the hare applies…a steady pace wins the race. If you try to push yourself too fast, you may be disappointed. I can give you an example from my own personal health. When I had candida, I decided to follow a protocol that required me to take simple steps every day. Instead of being inconsistent and going in spurts, I took a steady approach. My goal was to resolve the candida, not to end up with the same symptoms months later. In the end, it only took a short time for me to resolve the candida, but again, I was consistent and focused on following my protocol each day.

Whether I use this steady action approach on fitness goals, business goals or health goals, I've found that taking action and sticking to it — without expecting results too quickly — brings awesome results!

MASTERY — ONE STEP AT A TIME

Now that you understand the Five Principles of *High Raw*, you are ready to take action to master them! Now, challenges will show up along the way, no doubt about it. But this principle of taking action can help you work through challenges too! And in chapters 10–13, I have outlined success factors for getting started with your *High Raw* lifestyle, making it work for the long term and overcoming stumbling blocks.

The key to successfully taking action is to take one step at a time. You don't need to master everything at once. Imagine if you were trying to learn four new skills at once: tennis, skiing, knitting and running a successful carpet cleaning business. What do you think it would feel like if you had never done any of them and you expected to do well in all of them at once? It would be a disaster. But, let's say all four of these skills were your passion. You really loved cleaning carpets. You want to be the best tennis player on the planet. You want to be a great skier and you want to knit beautiful sweaters. How could you possibly accomplish all four of these skills? The only way to master so many new skills is to take one at a time, master it and move on to the next. This is what I'm inviting you to do with the Five Principles of *High Raw*. Take one and master it, then move on to the next.

The key is, continue to take action! Make each principle your monthly focus. Use what you learn from chapters 10–13 to support your journey. Most likely, you will find that with each step, you are feeling better and better until your health is transformed. Trust that mastering all of these is going to take you to the next level and that you have plenty of time to get there at your own pace. Remember, if your goal is to have FUN along the way, taking things one step at a time can keep the whole journey enjoyable.

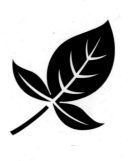

CHAPTER 10

GETTING STARTED: CREATING YOUR FOUNDATION FOR SUCCESS

The Five Principles of **High Raw:**

- PRINCIPLE #1: Eat Real Food & Think Like A Raw Foodist
- PRINCIPLE #2: Make Your Health Your TOP Priority
- PRINCIPLE #3: Know Your Body
- PRINCIPLE #4: Educate Yourself
- PRINCIPLE #5: Take Action!

Now that you understand the Five Principles of *High Raw,* how do you put them in action? In this chapter, you will learn how to create a foundation for *High Raw* so that you can get started successfully.

When you build a house, it is only as strong as the foundation. The same is true for your success in transforming your health. The process of any change is both physical and emotional. How you feel physically and emotionally can either help or hinder your success and in this chapter, you will learn tips and techniques for a strong foundation of physical and emotional health.

I highly recommend starting a *High Raw* journal to use along with this chapter because you will be doing some exercises and learning some new techniques to get started on your journey into the *High Raw* lifestyle. In any goal worth achieving, you will reach some stumbling blocks. There will be challenges and frustrations. This chapter will help you create such a strong vision and foundation for your health that it can keep you focused if challenges arise. If you feel you are going off track, this is where you can come to regroup and refocus.

HEALTH IS PHYSICAL AND EMOTIONAL

When it comes to the decision to get healthy, everyone starts in a different place. If you are feeling stuck, lazy, tired, angry, stressed out, anxious or upset, remember, it's not YOU. Your emotions are tied to your physical composition and chances are, as you clean up your physical body, your emotions will clean up as well.

Principle #1: Eat Real Food and Think Like a Raw Foodist is about following a largely plant-based diet. As you do this, you will find that your body begins to clean out. I like to think of it as cleaning a fish tank that was really dirty and full of algae. If you fill the tank with clean water, eventually, all of the dirt and algae will flush out of the top of the tank. Pretty soon, the tank will be clean. That's what's happening when you follow Principle #1. You're cleaning your internal body out so that your blood is alkaline and your body is balanced. You simply feel better, which boosts your moods and emotions.

So if you are starting from a place of feeling less than optimistic, remember — it's not you...it's not your soul or your interior. It's what's happening in your body that is creating how you feel.

We are meant to be enlightened, excited and energized beings. We are meant to be spiritual and to feel connected. As you follow Principle #1, your physical composition will improve and your energy will start to vibrate at a higher level. Once this happens, everything else begins to feel easier...everything starts to fall into place. You may find that you feel less stress and more excitement about each of the steps you are taking.

So what do you do in the meantime as your body is cleaning out? Can you still get started if you are not feeling emotionally optimistic about your goals for better health? Absolutely! That's what this chapter is all about. The ideas, techniques and exercises that follow will help you work with your mind and emotions, so that you can establish a mindset for success — one that supports you in achieving your physical health.

As you change the food you eat, you can also change the thoughts you think. Both of these actions will help "clean the fish tank," so to speak. So let's start first with getting to know your personality type.

GETTING TO KNOW YOURSELF — YOUR PERSONALITY TYPE

The first place to start in creating your foundation for success in the Five Principles of *High Raw* is to get to know yourself. This is a bit different from Principle #2: Know Your Body because this is about your personality type.

In my work as a personal trainer and health coach, I have noticed three personality types. Keep in mind that these are broad generalizations and not meant to pigeonhole anyone. This is not a complex discussion about Myers-Briggs Personality Type Indicators or the Enneagram. Instead, I want to share my observations about general personality types and how you can be successful no matter where you start.

The three personality types are:

- **PERSONALITY TYPE #1 — THE GO-GETTER**
  This person is very high energy and maybe even intense. The go-getter is a free spirit, has many interests and wants to dabble in all of them and has a hard time making a commitment. The go-getter has a lot of passion, is not afraid to take risks and may be inclined to be an entrepreneur. They tend to jump in and take action without needing to do much research.

- **PERSONALITY TYPE #2 — THE RESEARCHER**
  This person digs right in and does research before taking action. The researcher wants to know all the information up front before moving forward. The researcher tends to be more analytical and detailed, like an accountant, office manager or lawyer.

- **PERSONALITY TYPE #3 — THE CARETAKER**
  The caretaker is very heart-centered, compassionate and always looking out for other people. The caretaker is empathetic and cares deeply for other people and the planet. Often, caretakers give so much that they forget to take care of themselves. Some examples of caretakers might be a nurse, veterinarian or teacher.

As you read these three personality types, do you see yourself in one of them? Or perhaps you have different personality traits in different areas of your life? I know I do...for example, in my business, I am more of a go-getter — I jump in and I take risks. But when it comes to my health, I move a bit more into the researcher side – I'm still willing to take some risks, but I take it more slowly, do my two-week experiments and research more first.

Now which personality type do you think would be most successful at getting started with the *High Raw* lifestyle? As you can see, each of them have their strengths and weaknesses and that's true for all of us, isn't it?

The go-getters may seem like they'll just jump right in, but the danger is that they will move right on to something else, instead of sticking to their plan. They may not research enough to really understand what they need to do. The researchers may be really smart and learn a lot, but it may take them a long time to jump in and take action. And finally, the caretakers might find it difficult to take time for themselves because they are too busy caring for everyone else (but, they'll likely inspire a bunch of people to try it before them!).

So the key here is to take a little bit from each one of them, because chances are, we all have parts of ourselves that resonate with all three personality types. Which do you need to cultivate, in order to be successful?

If you're typically a go-getter, you may benefit from cultivating the researcher personality type so that you can learn more about nutrition and health. If you're a researcher, you can benefit from being more like the go-getter when it comes to taking action. And if you are a caretaker, you may want to turn that habit around and focus your caretaking on yourself, while cultivating more of the go-getter and researcher personality types.

How can you use this knowledge to improve your health? I recommend that if you are keeping a *High Raw* journal, that you write down which personality type you feel best describes your usual approach to health. Once you've done that, think about how you can benefit from one of the other personality types so that you can reach your goals.

If you are a researcher, I'd recommend you think about moving into a go-getter type mentality. What are some ways in which you could do that? If you could pick just one thing and say, "Hey, I'm going to jump in and do it and trust that everything will work" what would it be? Perhaps you can work with an expert, who has already done the research, so that you can take action faster. As a researcher, you may find that trusting someone else relieves the pressure of always having to figure things out for yourself.

If you are a go-getter, you might want to ask yourself, "What am I willing to research? What am I willing to commit to and for how long?" Give yourself time to allow results to show up. You might consider reading about the two-week experiments in chapter 7. You can also benefit from working with an expert who has done the research already, allowing you to keep moving forward.

If you are a caretaker, how will you put more time into taking care of yourself? You may feel that it's selfish at first, but that's just because you are more used to taking care of others. How can you be more like the go-getter?

No matter what your personality type, everyone can benefit from creating a success team that includes nutrition and health experts, along with a network of mentors, friends and family members who will share your interests and support you on your journey.

CREATING YOUR SUCCESS TEAM

The most successful people didn't get there by going it alone. In fact, if you talk to anyone who has achieved success from athletes to business people to artists, you will find that they had help along the way from a mentor, coach, teacher or expert.

In chapter 7, I talked about the importance of working with a health practitioner. If you are truly ready to make changes in your health, a health practitioner may be someone you want on your team. Who else would you include?

When creating your success team, the most important thing to consider is: who will help you on your journey?

Any goal worth achieving, including creating your best health, is going to have its rewards and its challenges. Often, it is during the challenging times that we tend to think about giving up. Your success team should include people who you can lean on or who will support and motivate you through the challenging times and of course, people who will celebrate with you during the good times.

Here are some options for your success team:

- HEALTH PRACTITIONERS
- FRIENDS
- MENTORS knowledgeable in health and nutrition
- FAMILY MEMBERS who are supportive of your health goals
- SUPPORT GROUPS working on related goals — these can be in-person, by phone or online

In general, you are looking for like-minded people who are ready to participate with you in your journey in some way. They may be providing advice, guidance and expertise or perhaps, simply an understanding ear when you need to talk. When you work with people who share your vision for your best health, it is a much richer journey.

If you are using a *High Raw* journal, make a list of the people you'd like to be on your success team. Take action by asking them to support you with your health goals!

CREATING YOUR VISION FOR YOUR BEST HEALTH

Now that you have a sense of your personality type and who you want on your success team, let's talk about creating your vision for your best health. When you write a vision, you are getting clear on what you want to create – on what you are passionate about creating. When you are passionate about something, you have a strong desire to make it happen.

Napolean Hill, author of *Think and Grow Rich* and one of the most influential people in the personal success movement said, "Desire is the starting point of all achievement, not a hope, not a wish, but a keen pulsating desire which transcends everything."

When you look at *High Raw* Principle #2: Make Your Health Your TOP Priority and *High Raw* Principle #5: Take Action, you can go much further if you have a vision of your best health...something you are passionate and excited about.

Here are two exercises to help you create a vision and passion for your health:

Exercise #1 - Linking Your Passion to Your Health

First, identify what you are truly passionate about when it comes to your health. I often hear goals like, "I want to have six-pack abs" or "I want to be 100% raw." These goals will certainly require several steps in order to achieve them, but it's not the series of exercises or types of foods that people want to hear about. Anyone can give you a series of steps to carry out your goals. Instead, I encourage you to understand what you are passionate about.

ASK YOURSELF THESE QUESTIONS:
- What am I doing right now? Do I like it?
- How do I want it to be?
- How do I want to feel?
- Once I achieve these goals, how will I feel?
- What makes me truly excited?
- What do I really like to do?

- What will make this fun for me?
- What am I really passionate about?
- What are my dreams?
- What motivates me?
- What's important to me?
- What am I doing when I feel my best?

The answers to your questions may have nothing to do with having six pack abs or being 100% raw. Maybe you're an accountant who really wants to be an Alpaca farmer. Or you're a nurse who wants to open a raw food restaurant. When I work with my clients, I always ask them what their dreams are — what they really want to do. I've found that when you get to the heart of what people really want, you can like that emotion to a healthier lifestyle.

How do you feel when you think about what really gets you juiced or excited?

It feels great doesn't it? Now think about doing a bunch of sit ups to get six pack abs…how does that feel in comparison? The truth is, what you are passionate about is much more inspiring than a bunch of tasks that you can carry out to meet your goals. Now don't get me wrong, the tasks are important too, but the first step is to know what you are passionate about and to link THAT to your goals for a healthy lifestyle.

So let's say you came to me and said you wanted to lose 10 pounds. After talking with you, I find out you're an accountant who really wants to be an alpaca farmer. As a personal trainer, I might talk to you about alpacas while you are doing some of your exercises. In this way, you will learn to associate good feelings with the behavior of exercise. There are many ways you can do this — be creative! If you love to be outside, you might start exercising by going for a hike instead of going to the gym.

One of my passions is climbing to the top of mountains and looking out at the view. So my wife, Annmarie, and I often hike for exercise. On a trip to Peru, we climbed up Mount Putukusi in the town of Aguas Calientes. Not knowing what to expect on this trail, we encountered a huge ladder that went along a cliff toward the top. There were actually several ladders that we later found out were considered "hair raising" in the guidebooks. As we were hiking, we watched many people decide to turn back, but we kept going. By the time we made our way around a big boulder at the top, we were amazed to see spectacular views of Machu Picchu.

This was literally one of the most beautiful experiences I've ever had. And I had to ask myself, "What if I wasn't so passionate about climbing mountains?" Surely, I may have turned back like so many others had. Instead, Annmarie and I stuck to our plan to get to the top and we felt tremendously rewarded. To me, the fact that we stuck to our plan and were rewarded with a view beyond our imagination was more spiritual than actually being at Machu Picchu!

You can do this too, by getting clear about what excites you – what you are passionate about – and then linking those good feelings with the steps you take toward your health goals. If you can associate those incredible feelings — of success, of feeling awesome, feeling love — to your exercise or to your health program, then it's going to make all the difference.

Exercise #2 — The Perfect Day

One of the most powerful things you can do for yourself to help you take action is the Perfect Day exercise. You can do it with any goal, whether about your health, your life, your relationships, your work or your family.

Start out by thinking about your most perfect day. What

would it be like? Now write down everything you can think of in detail.

Here are some things you may want to include:
- How would you wake up? Would the alarm go off? How would the sun come in?
- Who would you wake up with?
- What would you see or do when you wake up?
- What would you eat?
- How would you spend your day?
- Who would you spend your time with?
- What would you have for lunch?
- Who would you eat lunch with?
- How would you feel throughout the day?

Write everything down about your perfect day, from the time you wake up until the time you go to bed. Focus on how you feel as you write this and write that down too. Pay special attention to how you feel when you read and envision yourself in your perfect day. This is your vision of how you want your life to be. And how you feel as you visualize yourself in your perfect day is what I want you to "bottle up" and remember.

It is that feeling — how you feel in your perfect day — that is your catalyst for action and your motivator when things get tough. When you can connect to how you want to feel, it will support you in achieving your goals.

Once you write your vision for your perfect day, make a list of 15 actions you can take to move closer to your vision. Keep the action steps really simple. One example is that if your perfect day involves sitting on the beach and you are actually in the middle of a cold winter season, one action step might be booking a plane ticket for a beach vacation. If that's not possible, how about cutting out a picture of a beautiful, sunny beach and putting that on your bulletin board or finding a picture that you can save on your computer. These may seem simple, but they help bring the energy of that emotion closer to where you are right now. Each action step is designed to bring you a step closer to your vision of your perfect day.

Let's say you are currently experiencing chronic pain every day and your perfect day involves feeling great and being pain-free. What steps would you take to feel your best? While it might not be possible to become pain-free in one day, you could still write down some action steps, such as, "I'm going to research another possibility because maybe what I'm doing right now isn't working."

Whether it's a health goal or any other goal, we often can get stuck in a pattern of doing the same things over and over, while expecting a different result. Sound familiar? That's the definition of insanity and yet, I'm sure it's happened to all of us at times. We want to make a change, but we're not sure what to do differently.

Writing your perfect day vision can help you find creative ways to do things differently...because you will get really clear about the results you want to achieve and how you want to feel. Most of us are clear about what we DON'T want, instead of being clear about what we DO want. After you do this exercise, see if you come up with some creative actions you can take. Notice if you feel excited about the actions because they are linked to your passions and your dreams.

Once you complete the first 15 actions you've written down, come up with another 15 actions and move on from there. Don't be surprised if you look back after six months and find yourself feeling truly transformed!

When you think of failure, what comes to mind? Is it something you're afraid of? Does it keep you from taking risks or making changes? I believe that it's time to reframe failure from something terrible to something positive. What if you believed failure was a blessing? What if you trusted that if you failed, you would have learned a valuable lesson that would help you succeed in the future?

Thomas Edison had two years of failures before he invented the light bulb, but instead of quitting, he used the failures as learning opportunities. What if failure was a way to find a better way of doing something, instead of a reason for quitting?

If you believed failure was a blessing, a way to learn and an opportunity to grow, then you wouldn't be afraid of failure, would you?

In the book, *The New Psycho-Cybernetics*, by Dr. Maxwell Maltz, there's a great story about the mindset of failure.

Maltz describes going out for a hike...so put yourself into this scenario:[1]

Let's say you want to go for a hike, so you get some snacks and water and head out to a nature reserve. You park your car next to the tallest tree, which you'll use to identify how to get back from your hike.

The hike is the most amazing experience you've ever had...there are deer eating right from your hands and beautiful scenery. As you walk, many good ideas are coming to you, making you feel energized. You are snapped out of your reverie when it starts to get dark, so you begin to head back. As you spot the tree, you realize you've gone farther than you expected. But you know which direction to walk as you head back.

As you are walking, you begin going downhill and end up in a gully. As you look around, you don't recognize your surroundings. You've lost the trail and you're not sure where you are. As you look for the tree, you can't see it because you are too far down in the gully. Now you are starting to get scared...

So what do you do? Most people would curl up and sit there and sulk. They would say, "Oh man, I'm lost. I'm never going to get home. I don't even know where I am. Why did I even try this? That's it, I give up." They might simply sit and wait as it gets dark and cold. They may sink into worry, fear or stress. They may think they'll never find their car.

Another group of people will start to think about how to resolve the situation. Instead of giving up, their mind starts to ask questions like, "Well, how can I get out of here? How can I find my car?" As they look for solutions, they may look up and realize that because they are in a gully, they can't see the tree where they parked. They start thinking that if they could just walk to the top of the hill, they could look across the horizon and see the tree. So let's say you are one of these people. You walk to the top of the hill, you look out again and there's the tree. You're back on track. You start going. You get back before it gets dark. You get home and have dinner with your family. Everything's cool. Imagine how much further you'd be in your health path if you embraced failure like this?

Whether you are suffering from a serious illness or simply want to improve your health, if you focus on asking the right questions, like, "How can I get better? How can I find my dream? How can I reach my goal?", you're more likely to succeed every single time.

Another great metaphor comes from my days as a kid at the Bowlerama. Remember bowling as a kid? You got to use the lanes with those bumpers that kept your bowling ball from going into the gutter? As a kid bowling, I never had to worry about getting a gutter ball. Those bumpers gave kids a way to just relax and enjoy bowling — we could always get a pin or two to go down. If the ball got stuck, we could ask someone for help. We knew it would be okay.

What if you simply knew you would be okay when it comes to your health? What if you trusted that you could not fail and that you could ask for help if you needed it? What if you trusted that keeping it simple was all it took? That's what *High Raw* is about — a simple solution to feel your best. When you create the right mindset — creating a vision and passion for your health and trusting the steps you choose to take, you have everything you need to succeed.

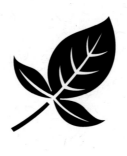

CHAPTER 11

MAKING IT WORK: YOUR TOOLBOX SYSTEM FOR SUCCESS

One of the best techniques I've found to help you take action successfully is the "Toolbox System." I introduced the toolbox system in my program, Seven Steps to Optimal Health When you set up your own Toolbox System, it can help you reach your health and wellness goals. In fact, you can use the Toolbox System for any of your goals.

Each of the tools in your Toolbox System is meant to help you take action. Anyone who has worked with me knows that I am a big proponent of systems. Why?

Systems help people take action successfully because they are:

- PROVEN: systems are created after much successful use from experts or through experience.

- REPEATABLE: systems allow you to have a set of activities you can use over and over again without reinventing the wheel.

- EASY: systems tend to be easy because they allow you to follow a process that has already been set up and organized.

The High Raw Toolbox System can help you achieve long-term success in your health and wellness goals. The four key toolbox systems are:

1. Fitness

2. Nutrition

3. Spiritual

4. On-the-Go

Toolboxes are also valuable because they give you a set of tools to make your work faster and easier. Imagine building a house...you have all the lumber and materials, you have your blueprint, but the only tool you have is a hammer. What would it be like trying to build a house with only one hammer? How would you saw the wood or paint the house?

Most likely, you'd take a trip to the hardware store and get a table saw, tile cutter, circular saw, screwdrivers, power drill, wire cutters, paint brushes — all the tools you need to build your house. Imagine how much easier that would be?

The Toolbox System gives you an organized set of options so that you can take action easily and quickly. Your Toolbox System is whatever you want to make it. It might be a set of folders with the information you need or a box with equipment you like to use. This is your opportunity to be creative — stock your Toolbox System with the materials you need to make your health and wellness goals easy. I am going to give you some suggestions to get things started and you can take in any direction that supports your goals.

GETTING STARTED WITH YOUR HIGH RAW TOOLBOX SYSTEM

While you can set up as many toolboxes as you like, my recommendation is that you start with four key categories: Fitness, Nutrition, Spiritual and On-the-Go.

FITNESS TOOLBOX

Your fitness toolbox will contain exercise options and tools. For this toolbox, I suggest you gather up some easy, fun fitness routines that you select from books or magazines. You may also want to include CDs, DVDs and equipment, like dumbbells, an exercise ball, a medicine ball or exercise bands. Be creative and include anything that helps you with your fitness goals. If cutting out pictures of fit people is motivating, do that. The idea is to keep your fitness toolbox organized and easily accessible for your regular use.

Here are some tips for your Fitness Toolbox:

You can add our easy-to-implement book on fitness called the Busy Person's Fitness Solution! This can be found at this address: www.gohighraw.com/bpfs

You can find a wide range of exercise equipment, bands, balls and more at Perform Better: www.gohighraw.com/performbetter

- FITNESS TOOLBOX TIP #1: *ORGANIZE.* Put your workouts and fitness plans into a 3-ring binder to keep them organized and easily accessible.

- FITNESS TOOLBOX TIP #2: *KEEP IT SIMPLE.* Whether you start with only one workout option or a few, keep it simple. There is no need to gather hundreds of workout options. Choose one that feels easy and start there, then add more exercises over time. A group of about 15 workout options can give you variety without being overwhelming as you are getting started. If you start to get bored, add more.

- **FITNESS TOOLBOX TIP #3:** *CHOOSE WORKOUTS YOU LIKE.* I love hiking, so I might put several hiking trails of different times (if I have 30 minutes or a couple hours, for example) in my fitness toolbox. I also like body-weight exercises, so I'd include several of those as well. Identify the workouts you like best and put several options into your fitness toolbox. Perhaps you will include some other options you'd like to experiment with as well.

- **FITNESS TOOLBOX TIP #4:** *BE FLEXIBLE FOR TIMING AND LOCATION.* How do you make this work, even when you are busy? Give yourself fitness options for different time frames and different locations. This way, if you can't workout outside or you can't make it to the gym, you have options for at-home fitness. The goal here is to make fitness a part of your regular lifestyle, so if your best laid plans for a given time frame or location go awry, you have other options you can use instead.

  When you select a group of workouts, include these options:
  - 10-minute workout
  - 15-minute workout
  - 30-minute workout
  - 60-minute workout

  For location, consider these options:
  - At the gym
  - Outdoors
  - Indoors

NUTRITION TOOLBOX

This one is fun and you may already be doing this to some degree already. To make your nutrition toolbox, gather up all of the cookbooks and recipes you have. Go through them and select the recipes that appeal to you. Then get all the recipes that you and your family would like and put

For ideas on bodyweight exercises, go to www.gohighraw.com/exercises. Here you will find 125 excellent exercise ideas that require no equipment. Each exercise has instructions and pictures so you can get started with your own fitness routine.

them into one binder. If you're like me, you'd rather not be sifting through 20 or more cookbooks to find the meal you want to make for dinner. Instead, when you get home from a long day, you have your binder within easy reach for your evening meal. Or maybe you already have a box of index cards with recipes — that works too!

Here are some tips for your Nutrition Toolbox:

- NUTRITION TOOLBOX TIP #1: *THINK VARIETY.* Give yourself a wide variety of options for meals, snacks and side dishes. Choose options that will allow you to experience a range of different foods and tastes, so that you keep things interesting when it comes to mealtime. As you experiment with new meals over a couple of months, you will get to see which meals are most appealing to you and your family.

- NUTRITION TOOLBOX TIP #2: *THINK TIMING.* You may want to put a marker on the recipes that are really fast – for those days when you are on the run. It's always helpful to have several options for a really quick meal. Make notes on the 5-minute and 10-minute meals so that you always have options, even at the busiest times.

- **NUTRITION TOOLBOX TIP #3:** *CONSIDER MENU PLANNING.* Consider planning the recipes you want to make each week and then making a grocery list of the foods you need ahead of time. Perhaps you simply want to have a section in your binder for "this week" and move the recipes you want to make into that section. This will make it easier to see what foods to buy when you are making your grocery list.

- **NUTRITION TOOLBOX TIP #4:** *MAKE EXTRA MEALS.* When you prepare meals, make extra. If you are making dinner, what about making extra so that you have something for the next day's meals? Or perhaps you'd like to take a day and make several meals that you can have on hand for the week. Your nutrition toolbox will have all the ideas you need to plan ahead.

SPIRITUAL TOOLBOX

This is my favorite toolbox. You don't need to be religious to have a spiritual toolbox. Think of this as your toolbox for inspiration and motivation. The focus is to find out what inspires you and makes you feel uplifted. When you feel inspired, it is energizing and when you are energized, you are more likely to continue forward with your goals.

Your spirituality toolbox might include a shrine of special pieces that motivate you. It could be something you keep in a corner of your room or at your desk. In this location, you'd put special objects that have meaning for you and that make you feel good. You might hang up collages with images that have powerful meaning to you. I keep my spiritual toolbox at my desk. On my desk, I have some rocks I had found from several special places. I also keep some silver pieces with insignias and books that have truly inspired me. Next to my desk, I have a collage with images that remind me of my vision.

If challenges arise on the way to reaching your goals (and they will!), you can go to your spiritual toolbox and spend time with the objects that inspire you. Perhaps you would do a meditation, prayers or mantras to clear your mind and heart. The act of visiting your spiritual toolbox can be very grounding and centering. It can bring you back to the part of you that is enthusiastic and positive about your life. It can help you forget the details of life and focus on the bigger picture.

Here are some tips for your Spiritual Toolbox:

- **SPIRITUAL TOOLBOX TIP #1:** *CHOOSE WHAT INSPIRES YOU.* This can be anything — books, CDs, DVDs, pictures, objects, prayers, meditations or mantras.

- **SPIRITUAL TOOLBOX TIP #2:** *CONSIDER MAKING YOUR SPIRITUAL TOOLBOX PART OF YOUR DAILY ROUTINE.* While your spiritual toolbox is there to lift your spirits if you are feeling down or feeling like you want to give up, consider visiting your spiritual toolbox daily or regularly, even when you are feeling great. A regular practice of focusing on what inspires you is very energizing.

- **SPIRITUAL TOOLBOX TIP #3:** *TRUST YOUR SPIRITUAL TOOLBOX AS A SELF-HELP TOOL.* Even if you aren't sure it will work, sit with your spiritual toolbox if you are really looking for help and don't know where to turn. Commit to sitting for at least five minutes and simply looking at or listening to some of the items in your spiritual toolbox. You may find that this is all you need to get you going in the right direction again and it can be very empowering to realize that you are your own best support!

We are all busy these days, so it helps to have options for those days you are really on the run. The on-the-go toolbox is your way of taking your healthy lifestyle with you wherever you are. Select a bag or box and fill it with the items you need for your health and fitness routine. For example, you might have a workout bag with running shoes, exercise clothes, some bottles of water and easy healthy snacks that don't need to be refrigerated (like trail mix).

Here are some tips for your On-the-Go Toolbox:

- ON-THE-GO TOOLBOX TIP #1: *MATCH YOUR ON-THE-GO TOOLBOX WITH YOUR LIFESTYLE.* Notice how you typically live your life — what do you find that you wish you had with you when it comes to meeting your health and fitness goals? Is it having healthy snacks on hand? Is it having your fitness gear with you so you can exercise during your lunch hour? When you are away from home, what will help you meet your goals? Stock your on-the-go toolbox with these items so that you are always prepared.

- ON-THE-GO TOOLBOX TIP #2: *KEEP IT SIMPLE.* Stick to necessities so that you don't feel overburdened with too many things.

- ON-THE-GO TOOLBOX TIP #3: *MAKE RE-STOCKING ROUTINE.* Think of your on-the-go toolbox as part of your routine. When you are grocery shopping, what snacks can you get to replenish your on-the-go snacks? When you are doing laundry, what exercise clothes do you need to wash and put into your on-the-go toolbox?

The toolbox system is all about preparation. You wouldn't build a house without any tools, right? That would seem kind of foolish. So it's just as important to have the tools you need when you are building a new routine around health and wellness. You don't have to wait until you have all of your toolboxes created or until they are all completely stocked — you can start now, but start with the goal of creating a toolbox system that will support you along the way.

Perhaps, like me, all you need to get started is one book. Mine was *The Seeker's Guide* by Elizabeth Lesser. One book is a good way to start taking action, but your toolbox system will help you stick with it over the long term.

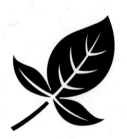

CHAPTER 12

THE MOST IMPORTANT PRACTICES BEYOND DIET

The food you eat is very important when it comes to creating a healthy *High Raw* lifestyle. However, diet is only one component of health and wellness. *If you want to achieve optimal health, the most important practices beyond diet are breath, water and exercise.* If you think about it in a hierarchy, if we stop breathing, we die in minutes. Without water, a person would feel adverse affects in one day and could possibly live up to 10 days depending upon other factors. Without food, it is estimated that humans could live for between four to six weeks. So while food is important, it is hardly the most important when it comes to your health.

As you approach your health and wellness goals, focusing on breath, water and exercise can help you feel your best.

BREATH

Depending upon several factors, you may not be breathing fully and completely. For example, are your clothes tight? Are you sitting at a desk all day? Are you feeling stressed out? Any of these things may keep you from taking full, deep breaths and nourishing your brain and body with the oxygen it needs to function properly.

If you want the easiest way to calm your mind and body, simply focus on taking deep, full and conscious breaths several times per day. Here's how:

- TUNE IN AND NOTICE IF YOU ARE TAKING SHALLOW BREATHS. Are you feeling constricted in any way? Sit or stand so that you can take deep, full breaths.

- ARE YOU BREATHING ALL THE WAY INTO YOUR BELLY? Focus on filling your entire body with air, all the way into your belly. Feel your belly expand with air.

- EXHALE DEEPLY AND FULLY.

- DO THIS FOR FIVE TO TEN BREATHS AND SEE HOW YOU FEEL. Take your time — even if you are feeling rushed, don't rush your breathing. The simple act of slow, deep breaths can be a signal to your whole body to slow down and feel more calm.

I've been focusing on this in my own life because I sit at a desk in front of a computer all day. Each day, I take time out to take full, deep, conscious breaths and it makes a big difference in how I feel. You might set a timer and do this a few times per day or wear a band on your wrist to remind you to take deep, conscious breaths. Experiment with this for two weeks and see if you feel calmer and less stressed. You may even find that you feel more energized.

WATER

Your body is made up of 75% water and your brain is made up of 90% water, so you can imagine how important it is to hydrate your body. Unfortunately, our planet has very polluted water. Humans have polluted many of our clean water sources and taken the life out of the water we drink. The result of all of this pollution is tap water that is cleaned with chemicals, which are also harmful to the human body. In fact, there are so many ways of treating water just to make it drinkable, that it's hard to tell what affects it will have on human health.

So how do we get fresh, pure water? Not everyone lives near a fresh spring, where they can fill up bottles with pure water that has been tested as drinkable. The most realistic solution is to get some sort of filter, even if you have well water.

To find out how to get the best drinking water, go to www.RenegadeWaterSecrets.com and learn what the top health and water experts recommend!

Water Filters

Water filters are a great way to remove contaminants from tap water and well water. Some examples of contaminants are: heavy metals like lead, mercury and cadmium or additives like fluoride and chlorine. Water can also be contaminated by: pesticides, microorganisms, and even toxins from pharmaceutical drugs and personal care products.[1]

I have always been interested in finding the best sources of pure drinking water, which is why I researched and produced a program called Renegade Water Secrets. In Renegade Water Secrets, I gathered five of the world's top health and water experts and asked them to reveal their best techniques to getting clean, pure drinking water for your health and for the planet. After interviewing the experts, I found that the best water filter you can get is a reverse osmosis system. While it is a little wasteful in terms of water itself, it will give you the best drinking water and the good news is, they are not that expensive. Some of the reverse osmosis water filters are only about $300.

If you can't start out with a reverse osmosis water filter, start with something that fits your budget. The first place to start is with a filter that removes chlorine. An option for this type of filter is the Brita brand water filter, which has many options in a variety of price ranges. Eventually, you may want to upgrade your water filter to one that removes more of the common contaminants in water. The key is to start with what you can afford and then upgrade when you can.

I started with an Aqauasana water filter and upgraded from there. The next time I move, I'll upgrade to a reverse osmosis water filter. The key with water filters and every-thing else with respect to your health is to go at your own pace. This means go at the pace of your budget as well. When you can trust that with each upgrade, you are receiving more benefits, it's much more successful than being stressed about not having everything right now. That's what's called getting better. That's the process of mastery. Right now my water mastery is at a level that I would say is A minus and I'm committed to working on it, while at the same time, being satisfied with where I am right now. Remember, good health is physical and emotional, so the more you are happy about where you are right now, the easier it will be to move to the next level.

Shower filters are also important because your skin is your largest organ and it absorbs chlorine and other toxins from water. When you get into the warm shower, the pores in your skin open up, so you can imagine how chemicals from water can get into your body.

Alkaline Water

Depending upon the source of your water, it could be slightly acidic or slightly alkaline. Now you've heard me and possi-bly other experts talk about creating a more alkaline condi-tion in your blood to achieve optimal health, so you may be tempted by alkaline water systems. The idea behind alkaline water systems is that if you drink alkaline water, your body will absorb it and it will become more alkaline. I'm not completely sold on this, however.

While your blood should be slightly alkaline for your best health, the rest of your body is naturally either acidic or more alkaline. Your stomach is naturally acidic — it needs to be so that it can digest your food. When you drink alkaline water, your body will buffer the acidity so that it can stay at a neutral pH of 7.

If your stomach becomes less acidic, you will be less able to digest. This is why you would not want to take an antacid before you eat or why you would not want to drink alkaline water before you eat.

To find how you can get some of these products at a great discount, you can visit www.gohighraw.com/healthproducts

I think that adding some sea salt to your water can help to make it more alkaline, without having to invest in an alkaline water system. Sea salt is very alkaline and helps to balance the body's pH levels.

Hydration

Access to pure water for drinking and showers is important, but it's also critical to focus on how much water you are drinking. We are chronically dehydrated as a population too. So even if you think that you're drinking a lot of water, you're probably not drinking enough. *In Your Body's Many Cries For Water*, Dr. Fereydoon Batmanghelidj suggests that chronic dehydration may be the cause of conditions such as angina, migraines, hypertension, high cholesterol, chronic fatigue syndrome, MS, depression, arthritis and diabetes in the elderly.[2]

Drinking enough water is important, but absorbing the water you drink is also critical.

Symptoms of Dehydration:[3]

- Headache
- Dizziness or lightheadedness
- Fatigue
- Cravings
- Muscle Weakness
- Dark urine
- Few or no tears when crying
- Dry skin
- Thirst
- Dry mouth

Here are some tips for how to drink and absorb more water:

- ADD SEA SALT TO YOUR WATER. Adding a pinch of sea salt to your water is a great way to add minerals to your water.

- ADD LEMON TO YOUR WATER. Lemons have flavor and detoxification properties that make a great addition to your water.

- DRINK PLENTY OF WATER IN THE MORNING. Drink at least a liter of water (33 ounces), depending upon your size. When you wake up, your body is dehydrated, so drinking plenty of water will rehydrate your body and help with elimination.

- PUT A BIG GLASS JUG OF WATER AT YOUR DESK OR CLOSE TO WHERE YOU ARE WORKING. Having easy access to a jug of water is a great way to make sure you will drink plenty of water during the day.

- DRINK HALF YOUR BODY WEIGHT IN OUNCES OF WATER EACH DAY. This will help ensure you are drinking plenty of water.

- DRINK GREEN JUICES. I am convinced that green juices are the best thing on the planet. Experiment with drinking green juices yourself and see if you get an amazing boost of energy. I've found that green juices make my eyes feel open and provide longer lasting energy than just about anything else.

In order to drink enough water, you're likely going to want to carry your water around with you. If carrying a glass jar doesn't work for you, consider moving to stainless steel water bottles instead of plastic. Klean Kanteen is a brand of stainless steel water bottles that I like because they do not leach chemicals like plastic water bottles. Bisphenol A (BPA) is a toxin found in some plastics that has been found to be a hormone disruptor because it mimics sex hormones.

For good pricing on Stainless Steel water bottles like Klean Kanteen, you can visit this link: www.gohighraw.com/kleankanteen

It's important for you to decide how you want approach removing toxic exposure. Even if you are a purist in only one thing, it can still benefit from you. The idea is not to live your life stressed out about toxins. Instead, choose the areas in your life where you want to take a more pure approach because the steps you take in that area are going to reduce your toxic burden and boost your health.

When it comes to water, you might decide to focus only on removing mercury, chlorine and fluoride. That step alone will reduce your toxic load, which will benefit your health. Over time, you may take additional steps, trusting that with each new level, you continue to boost your health.

EXERCISE

I believe that exercise is just a little bit more important than food. When I look at people who have been exercising over a long period of time, I notice that they always look better. And I've also done a little experimenting myself with this whole idea of food and exercise. I started with exercise...it was "my thing." Way before I got into nutrition, I was committed to regular exercise. As I learned about nutrition, I became so food-centered that I stopped exercising for a while and my health started to suffer. That's when I realized that good nutrition and exercise together make a more well-rounded approach to good health.

When you exercise, what you're doing is wringing out your system. You are moving your lymph, which is one of your systems of detoxification. Exercise also helps your body remove toxins.

As your muscles contract, as you move your limbs and as you bounce, you're getting your entire system in motion. I believe the human body was made to move. When people tell me that they don't like to exercise, I am certain that they simply haven't found the exercise that is right for them. What makes most people dislike exercise or fail at exercise is that they don't like the exercise they are doing. Whenever I see this, I tell them to stop doing that exercise and find something they really like. When you are doing exercise you don't like, you are basically forcing yourself to do something that feels unpleasant – this means you are relying on willpower to get you through. It's much more successful to do something out of feeling empowered, rather than using willpower. I'll cover more on willpower vs. empowerment in chapter 13.

If you could go out and absolutely love the exercise you are doing, what would it be? Since I love to hike, I get out and climb mountains, look at the view and sit and eat wild foods. Because I love what I'm doing, it doesn't even feel like exercise. Instead, I'm having the time of my life and my exercise feels like play. Your goal is to experiment and find out what type of exercise you would really enjoy.

The Importance of Vigorous Exercise

One thing to keep in mind when it comes to exercise is intensity. I believe that vigorous exercise is essential. Yoga is great — it's very relaxing and meditative, but it serves a different purpose than vigorous exercise. Vigorous exercise would include high intensity or cardiovascular exercise. High intensity exercise is anerobic, which uses muscle sugar (glycogen) and cardiovascular exercise is aerobic, which uses oxygen. While either one of these are good to do, I recommend doing both as part of your fitness routine. Running, fast walking, jumping and hiking are great types of vigorous exercise.

While some people recommend a rebounder, I don't believe you get the best results in terms of exercise as a whole because it does not wring your muscles like other types of exercise. I always recommend choosing exercise that pumps your blood, moves your limbs and wrings your muscles.

Exercise and the Great Outdoors

Whenever possible, go outside for your exercise. When you are outside, you breathe in negative ions, which give you a positive mood. Additionally, the sun has vitamin D, which boosts your health and your mood. Next time you exercise outdoors, notice how you feel. The act of exercising outdoors is often enough to energize, recharge and revive you.

Exercise and Body Type

In Ayurvedic medicine, there are three different body types, called doshas. Each dosha has different physical and psychological characteristics. Each person's body type is a unique expression of a dosha or combination of the doshsas. You can find out your dosha by going to an Ayurvedic practitioner, but you can also look at general characteristics and identify which dosha you think you might be.

The three doshas in Ayurvedic medicine are: vata, pitta and kapha. Once you know your dosha, the practice of Ayurveda involves aligning your food, habits and lifestyle in a way that keeps your dosha balanced. The idea is that if you are balanced, you achieve health and wellness.

You can do the same thing with your exercise. Once you

know your dosha, you can choose an exercise routine that keeps you balanced. For example, the pitta dosha is firey and tends to get hot easily, while the vata and kapha doshas are much cooler. So how would you apply this knowledge to exercise?

Here are some guidelines for exercise and your dosha:

- **VATA DOSHA:** Consider an exercise that warms up this cooler body type, such as walking or dancing. Vatas tend to get stressed and worn out easily, so yoga can also be a good addition to your exercise routine.

- **PITTA DOSHA:** This intense, fiery dosha may want to do a cooling exercise, like some slow cardiovascular exercise. Since pitas tend to be competitive, playing sports may keep them engaged.

- **KAPHA DOSHA:** This slow, cooler dosha may benefit from a routine, warming and stimulating exercise, like weight lifting, tennis or running.

Pain and Joint Health

If you have pain in your joints, like knees, elbows, fingers and wrists, you can really benefit from exercise. This is not a "no pain, no gain" kind of mentality — that is old school. Instead, it's important to understand some of the reasons why exercise can help reduce or eliminate pain.

First of all, most of your joints are surrounded by a thick fluid, which helps them move. Called synovial fluid, this liquid actually helps you move painlessly and it also bathes your cartilage in nutrients. Think of synovial fluid as the WD40 for your bones and cartilage — it keeps things moving.

If you have painful joints or an arthritic condition, moving those joints actually helps them feel better, even if you think it would be the opposite. But clearly, you want to bring some pain relief to your joints so you can feel good while you exercise, so I'd like to share some good options for pain relief. First, arthritis and joint pain are inflammatory conditions, so reducing inflammation and acidic blood is important. I will cover more about how to reduce acidity in chapter 16. Keep in mind that if your blood is acidic, your synovial fluid may also be acidic, which means your cartilage is not getting the nutrients it needs. You can nourish your joints by creating an alkaline environment in your blood, staying well hydrated and supplementing with vitamin C, sulfur or MSM. This will help to build strong, healthy joints and connective tissue.

Another option for pain relief in sore joints is hot/cold therapy. Get a bucket of cold water and add some ice so that it's really chilled. Then get a bucket and fill it with water that is almost too hot to touch. Put the painful joint into the cold bucket for one minute and then put the joint into the hot bucket. Continue to alternate between hot and cold. You could do this in the shower for your knees, alternating between hot and cold water. Hot/cold therapy functions as a pump. The cold water contracts your capillaries and the hot water dilates them, so it's like wringing the blood and fluid out and then bringing it back in again. It's a great therapy for ankle sprains, knee issues, wrist problems and carpal tunnel conditions. It eliminates stagnation that is in your joints, in areas that may be building up toxins or waste products that you want to release.

TRANSFORMATION IS A STEP-BY-STEP PROCESS

While a healthy diet, breath, water and exercise are very important, you don't need to add all of these to your routine at once. Remember that transforming your health at your own pace is more important that making changes overnight.

I highly recommend that you create a calendar with your

goals and decide what you're going to do in a year, in five years and in ten years. Identify which new habits are important to you and decide when you will add each of them to your regular routine. Health doesn't have to mean you are a new person by tomorrow. Health is about creating good habits over a lifetime, so decide what works for you and plan it out accordingly.

CHAPTER 13

OVERCOMING POTENTIAL STUMBLING BLOCKS

Anytime you set goals or start taking action toward a big change in your life, you will experience challenges or stumbling blocks along the way. To understand this, let's use an example of driving to a job you've had for 10 years. Think about your commute to and from work — have you ever had one of those days where you get home and realize you don't remember driving from work to home at all?

The reason is that your trip is so ingrained in your mind that you don't even have to think about it anymore. If you encountered a detour one day and had to take a new route home from work, you'd actually have to think about which roads to take...you'd really have to pay attention. But for your usual trip home from work, it's so automatic that it seems like you barely have to pay attention...you're on autopilot.

It's the same with our habits. They are so ingrained that we are literally on autopilot as we go through our day. When you decide to change your diet, experiment with new recipes or start a new exercise routine, it may take some thought and planning at first. When everything is going well, you may find that doing things differently is pretty easy, but when stumbling blocks show up, it may feel more challenging.

Typical stumbling blocks on the way to creating your best health are: cravings, stress, information overload and feeling like you don't have the money to invest in the healthy food, products or services you desire. These stumbling blocks are so common that I receive hundreds of questions about them on a regular basis.

The first place I start in helping clients overcome stumbling blocks is the idea of willpower vs. empowerment.

WILLPOWER VS. EMPOWERMENT

Willpower is defined as self-control or controlling one's actions or impulses. It is what we are told we need to have in order to change our habits. Stephen Covey describes habits as having a "strong gravitational pull" in *The Seven Habits of Highly Effective People*. So if you think about it, when you apply willpower to change habits, it is a constant battle of the gravitational pull of that habit against your own forces of self-control.

Imagine what it feels like to be in a constant battle. You may do well at first, constantly pushing and pushing, but eventually, willpower crumbles. And when it does, you might simply go back to your old habit, feeling that it's the more powerful force. Humans both desire and resist change. While change may be desired, resistance to change is almost an instinctual way to protect ourselves. Resistance to change is a common reaction because humans tend to want things to remain in homeostasis or balance, which can often translate into to wanting things to stay the same. In fact, resistance to change is so strong that the fields of change management and organizational development were created to help organizations reach big goals by helping employees adapt to change.

So how can you change successfully so that you can reach

your health and wellness goals? Instead of focusing on the battle of willpower, imagine what it would be like to feel empowered? To be empowered means that you are equipped with ability or enabled. Think for a moment about the difference between imposing self-control to do something vs. feeling equipped and enabled to do something?

Juice Feasting expert David Rainosheck created the concept of the Spectrum of Diet™, which approaches diet and nutrition along a continuum from low life-force foods to high life force foods. The idea is that you can see where you are on the spectrum and work to move up to a more healthy way of eating. If you looked at the spectrum and you were eating a standard American diet (SAD), you'd see that you have many steps in the spectrum to go before you got to the raw food diet. Now, what I don't agree with here is putting food in a hierarchy, saying that the raw food diet is the best, but I do like the idea of seeing how you might progress from one type of eating to another. For example, if you are currently eating SAD, the progression would be to whole foods, then you might move to a vegetarian diet, then a plant-based diet and then to the raw food plant-based diet.

In other words, the Spectrum of Diet™ is showing the possibility of how you might progress. What if you felt you had to go from SAD to raw overnight? You'd be skipping several steps. You'd actually miss the skill, knowledge and behavior changes you might be making along the way. You might apply willpower to make the change and "bam," you'd be going from eating Twinkies to eating kale and drinking green smoothies. However, having skipped all the steps in between, you haven't really empowered yourself — equipped yourself with the ability to make the change. You might find that you have to grit your teeth and force yourself to stay on track.

Many people do this...they use willpower to go from

SAD to raw, without empowering themselves with the skills, knowledge and behaviors to really support a true change of habits. This is why so many people go right back to eating Twinkies again. Willpower eventually breaks down, and the timing is different for each person.

My goal in encouraging a step-by-step approach through the *Five Principles of High Raw*, is for you to equip yourself with the ability to create new healthy habits at your own pace. This is not an overnight switch, but a progression. If you say, "I'm going to do this" and slowly move up the ladder toward your goals, you can decide how you will move along the continuum toward a more plant-based diet as described in Principle #1: Eat Real Food and Think Like a Raw Foodist.

I recommend that you plan to make small adjustments from where you are now to where you want to be, unless there is a pressing health reason to make big, immediate changes. If your health requires big changes immediately, your health practitioner can be a great support in making a quick transition. For everyone else, there is really no need to make drastic changes. Remember that humans resist change, but you and your body may not even notice small changes. You give yourself a chance to get used to the change and then you build from there. This is a great way to coax yourself into making big changes over time. In a way, these small changes trick you into thinking that this is how you've been doing it all along.

If I had gone directly from SAD to raw food, I would still think about foods that I used to eat. I would still crave Entenmann's cake from the grocery store. Today, I don't crave those foods anymore and the thing is, it's because I know it isn't even food. I gave myself a chance to progress and learn over time.

When you aren't focused on being 100% raw or 100%

perfect, you'll see that you have the ability to move along the continuum of healthy eating all the time. If you are not feeling like having raw food, you might have steamed kale and cooked quinoa. You no longer have to bounce back and forth from one end of the spectrum to the other because you have learned how to support yourself with healthy eating along a continuum. You don't have to say, "If I failed at raw foods, I'll go back to pizzas, soda and Twinkies."

So when you're trying willpower it's never going to work. You're never going to be able to push yourself long enough because eventually it's going to crack. Instead, trust that you are empowering yourself to make changes in your life by building upon what you've learned before.

ELIMINATE CRAVINGS

Everyone has experienced cravings, but did you ever think about where the craving is coming from? Do you think it's you who doesn't have the willpower? Cravings are really a habit. In essence, you have associated a food with a feeling or emotion. From a physiological perspective, your body is looking for a hit of dopamine, sometimes called the "master molecule of addiction."

Dopamine is a neurotransmitter (chemical messenger) in your brain that is associated with the feeling of pleasure. When you eat a food you are craving, it stimulates dopamine, which then makes you feel emotions of happiness, satisfaction, reward or pleasure. The more concentrated a food (the more processed it is), the more you may stimulate dopamine, which is why many people have cravings for junk food. So YOU are not your cravings...in fact, you are responding to a chemical reaction in your body. There are other physiological reasons you may have cravings, but the dopamine reaction explains why your emotions may be so involved.

Are cravings making you feel like a zombie walking to the refrigerator? Are they sabotaging your goals to lose weight or maintain a healthy weight? It would be pretty tough to use willpower to overcome a physical and emotional reaction, wouldn't it?

I used to experience the pull of cravings myself. I used to host an open mic in Bethel, Connecticut every other Thursday. On those Thursday nights, I'd show up, play a couple of songs on my guitar and then invite everyone else up. People would sign up and play songs — and everyone would have a good time. It was at a coffee shop and they had the most incredible brownies. So I would have a brownie every Thursday night.

The thing is, I would get home and I wouldn't be able to sleep because the sugar in the brownies was intense. I would roll around in bed, wishing I never ate the brownie. In the morning, I'd wake up with dark spots under my eyes. I'd feel so tired that it was hard to get out of bed. In spite of how I felt, I would still go to the open mic and get a brownie every Thursday night.

One day, I made a decision, "I don't want to be addicted to these brownies anymore." But that didn't do a thing to stop the craving. I would sit down at the open mic and start playing a song...all the while, thinking about whether or not I was going to have a brownie. How ridiculous is that? It's a brownie...just a little piece of cake! It had this magnetic pull on me that was literally insane. But I knew that I needed to take control.

I realized one thing about myself when it came to brownies: I had this electrical charge towards them. There was something that was putting me in this position and giving me a feeling that I wanted. *I realized that if I could eliminate that charge, I wouldn't have to think about brownies any more.*

It's the same with any type of addiction. Think about cigarettes right now. If you are not a cigarette smoker, do you ever have a craving for cigarettes? Most likely you do not crave them at all. I used to be a cigarette smoker and when I was smoking cigarettes, I would crave them like crazy. Once I quit smoking and eliminated that craving, I have a whole different reaction to cigarettes. Today, if you put a pack of cigarettes in front of me — or even lit one and put it in my mouth, I would feel nauseous. I think it's disgusting. So what happened between craving cigarettes and not craving them? *I lost the emotional charge towards it.* I was able to replace it with something else.

Willpower just didn't work...making the decision alone didn't work.

Here's what does work for eliminating the charge of cravings:

- RECOGNIZE THAT CERTAIN FOODS ARE AN ADDICTION. Now that you understand the dopamine connection, you can see why certain foods, particularly foods high in sugar, are addictive. Instead of beating yourself up for having no willpower, you may decide not to eat addictive substances. More and more studies are showing how highly addictive sugar is. The only difference between sugar and cocaine, is that sugar is legal and readily available. Because sugar is so widely accepted and in so many processed foods, it causes many health issues. And it's not just processed sugar. You may find yourself addicted to other sweeteners because they have the same or a similar effect. I'll cover more about sweeteners in chapter 14.

  If you aren't sure about the addictive nature of sugar or other foods you are craving, pay attention to how you feel after you eat it. Do you feel hung over? Do you have dark circles under your eyes? I know that if I go to a restaurant and have any sort of sugar by mistake, like dressing in a salad or something, my body immediately reacts.

- **CLEAN OUT YOUR CUPBOARDS.** If you have food in your cupboard that you would rather not be eating, throw it out. Don't even bring it into the house. Let's say you want to avoid chocolate, but you keep a little stash in your house for when cravings strike. Think about what happens when you know a food you crave is in the house. You might be more likely to eat it. Instead, do not have these foods in your house.

- **ASK QUESTIONS.** Remember what got me on track with my health? I asked myself a question, "Is there something better than this?" You can do the same thing with cravings. Questions are very powerful because they get you out of autopilot and get you thinking differently. Ask yourself why you feel this pull. When I realized I was still craving brownies, I began to ask myself, "Why am I feeling this pull to these brownies?"

- **FIND OUT WHAT IS MISSING IN YOUR LIFE AND ADD SOMETHING BETTER.** Have you heard that craving sugar means you lack sweetness in your life? Cravings can often be distractions from what we really want in our lives. Think about what happens when you eat the food you are craving. When you eat sugar, do you feel warmth, peace or euphoria? Where are you missing those emotions in your life? What could you be doing that would allow you to experience them without food? The exercises in chapter 10, linking your passion to health and the perfect day exercise, are great ways to help answer these questions.

Let's use the cigarettes and brownies as an example in my

own life. What did cigarettes bring me? What do brownies bring me? In the case of cigarettes, I used them to breathe, relax, to be social, to take a break. I used brownies to have fun and to get a little pick-me-up.

Think about it, if you can identify why you're going towards the food you are craving, you can start to substitute it with something else that will give you a similar feeling. When I used to smoke cigarettes at work I would go and take a five-minute break, sit outside and have a cigarette. That's a nice break. Why couldn't I just go and sit outside and not have a cigarette? Why not? Or what if I took a five-minute break and did deep breathing, to give me more of what I was getting from the cigarette? Once you realize the payoff you are getting from any habit or craving, you can start to choose a healthier habit that fulfills what you truly want.

With the brownies, once I asked myself why I was so pulled to them, I finally said, "I get it." I decided to have a cup of herbal tea instead. I realized the tea would calm me and I wouldn't have to worry about the brownies anymore. How cool is that? So I completely eliminated that addiction to brownies.

- CREATE A PATTERN INTERRUPT. As you go through the process of eliminating cravings, you may recognize a pattern. A pattern interrupt is putting something between you and what you are craving so that instead of having the craving and then taking action by eating what you are craving, you do something to interrupt the act of eating.

  Let's use me and the brownie as an example. Let's say that I was craving a brownie. Instead of just eating it, I started drinking herbal tea. That interrupted my pattern of being on autopilot and just eating the brownie.

There are many options for pattern interrupts: repeat a mantra, do a meditation, go for a walk, call a friend or even the practice of asking yourself questions. A good question is, "Is there something better that I can reach for now?"

Just the simple act of asking yourself this question can help you change your habits. You can train yourself to reach for better things. When you go to the refrigerator at night and you're looking for something sweet and you ask yourself, "Is there something better that I can reach for?" You might end up having a salad. You can literally save yourself from the clutches of some sort of awful addiction that feels like it's controlling you — because you are empowering yourself to move beyond it and create new habits.

You can find out how to prepare some of these healthy snack ideas like kale chips on our website: www.RenegadeHealth.com

- CREATE A HEALTHY RECIPE INSTEAD. Anytime you change your diet, you may have tastes you miss. One example is crunchy food. The standard American diet is full of chips, pretzels and other crunchy snacks. The thing is, you can replicate many of the tastes you like with healthier versions of those foods. This may take some planning if you want to make it yourself. There are many recipe books that show you how to make meals that taste like foods you may have left behind. For crunchy foods, you could make raw crackers or chips, for example. You'd be surprised at how delicious crackers made with raw vegetables, nuts and seeds can be. Some examples are flax crackers or kale chips. You can even dip kale chips in raw tahini.

These snacks are really easy to make on your own, but if you don't have the time, there are some excellent options at the health food store or online raw food stores for raw chips and snacks made with healthy, organic ingredients. Going to a raw food restaurant, like Quintessence in New York City, is also a great way to sample healthy food. Quintessence makes amazing raw, non-GMO corn chips that will show you the potential you have to make delicious, healthy substitutions for junk food.

Remember to ask yourself questions first though. Is it crunchy food you are craving or is it really the salt? I think it's often the salt we're addicted to. As you eat a more plant-based diet, you may find that your body is getting more minerals and you won't crave salt as much.

So remember, instead of remaining in autopilot or that zombie phase of cravings, practice these techniques. You'll see that you become more conscious and aware of what's happening in your mind and body — and you'll be empowered to make real changes in your life.

Another important area to address with respect to eliminating cravings and reaching your health and well-being goals is reducing stress. Who of us isn't stressed out these days? Stress is a fact of life, but how you deal with it makes all the difference when it comes to your health.

REDUCE STRESS

Besides the typical aspects of life, we are bombarded with e-mail, the Internet and cell phones — sometimes, it may seem like we have too much to process in too little time. The fight or flight response of stress is meant to protect us in times of danger. However, many of us are feeling stress so often that it becomes chronic. Too much stress means too much cortisol, a hormone called the stress or death hormone. Elevated cortisol is linked to many health conditions, such as weight gain, premature aging, fatigue, lowered immunity and constipation.

Type A personalities, who are very driven, may react to stress more often than type B personalities, who are more laid back. As a type A personality, I know how critical it is to reduce stress. But the first thing you need to do is figure out what's causing the stress in the first place.

Just like with cravings, if you can identify what is causing the electrical charge, then you can get to the heart of what is causing stress. Let me give you an example. Let's say that you hear your company is going to have layoffs. You are having lunch with two friends and one of them is worrying about losing her job. She's wondering how she'll pay her bills and how long it will take her to find a new job. She's worrying about her family. Your other friend has decided that she's going to wait and see what happens, but she's also planning to update her resume, thinking perhaps this is an opportunity for an exciting new job. Which friend do you think is experiencing more stress?

How you react to any given situation determines the level of stress you will feel. Certainly, news of an impending layoff could cause stress, but the friend who immediately starts thinking of all the bad things that could happen is bound to feel more stress than the friend who is seeing a potential opportunity for change.

Two people can be in exactly the same situation and perceive it differently. Is it possible that a layoff could be equally perceived as scary and negative or exciting and positive? How you perceive any given situation is the key to the level of stress you experience.

For you, losing a job could have an electrical charge — or an emotional charge to it. Ask yourself, "What is it?" Are you worried about not being able to pay the bills...or not being able to survive? Often, at the very deepest level, stress has to do with survival — because it's a deeply ingrained, reptilian response to protect us and help us survive. Because it's reptilian, it comes from the part of your brain that is instinctual and automatic. However, you don't have to simply react in an automatic way to stress. If you pay attention and ask yourself questions during times of stress, you can decide how you want to perceive and respond to stressful situations.

Here are some techniques to reduce stress:

- **ASK QUESTIONS.** You've heard me suggest this technique again and again and for good reason: it helps remove you from unconsciously reacting in autopilot and instead, consciously responding to what is happening. Ask yourself what the electrical charge is to a particular stressful situation and then ask yourself, "How do I want it to be?" This will get you thinking about how to take action.

- **TAKE ACTION.** Taking a *High Raw* approach, think about Principle #5: Take Action. Once you have identified the electrical charge and how you really want it to be instead, you can start taking action to move in that direction. Let's say you've realized you are stressed about the lay-off because you're afraid you won't be able to pay your bills. How do you want it to be? Perhaps you decide that you want to feel comfortable that you can pay your bills and find a new job. So what action could you take? Maybe you decide to create a budget, so you can understand your expenses. Then you take a look at your savings and see how you are doing. And finally, maybe you put a spending plan in place that you feel comfortable with. You might even join your friend in updating your resume and looking for a new job. In fact, if your current job isn't the job of your dreams, perhaps you do the exercises in chapter 10 to identify your passion and your perfect day. What if you took action and found an even better job that you truly loved? Or started your own business that you had been dreaming about?

- Use stress relief techniques. We talked about pattern interrupts with respect to eliminating cravings and they can be excellent for stress relief as well. You could repeat a mantra, do a meditation, practice deep breathing, do yoga or anything that helps to calm your body and mind. I like using Emotional Freedom Techniques (EFT). EFT is a process of tapping on emotional acupuncture meridians, while repeating statements about releasing what you don't want and reframing what you do want. People have used EFT as a pattern interrupt and behavioral change for all kinds of issues from addictions to phobias and unwanted patterns. While I don't think it's a cure-all, I do think that tapping on those emotional acupressure points can help your mind and body relax.

  When you are stressed, notice what's happening in your body. Chances are, your breathing becomes shallow, your heart is beating faster and your muscles are tight — particularly in your neck and shoulders. EFT is great because it's easy and you can do it anywhere. If you are stressed, you may not be able to calm your mind and body enough to meditate or do yoga. With EFT, it's very active and actually acts as a bridge from a very stressed mind to a calmer, relaxed state.

- Notice if you are addicted to stress. You can become

addicted to stress, just like you can become addicted to sugar and other foods. This is often referred to as the "adrenaline lifestyle." One of the hormones secreted in the stress response is adrenaline, which gives you a shot of energy. That's what allows people to run really fast if they are being chased. Too much adrenaline, just like too much cortisol, is harmful for your body over time. However, just like an addiction to caffeine, you could become addicted to that hit of energy. Pay attention and see if this is true for you and if so, commit to actively reducing stress with the techniques mentioned here — or pick something else that works for you. Consider doing a two-week experiment with a low stress or low adrenaline lifestyle and seeing how you feel. Remember that this is a habit and it may take time to change. You may want to add this to your health goals and take steps toward making changes. If you are an adrenaline junkie, you might be someone who tries to take action on everything at once, which is exactly the opposite of what I am recommending in the *High Raw* approach. You owe it to yourself to find out how it feels to take things at a slower pace and enjoy the journey.

OVERCOME PLATEAUS

The term plateau is bandied about in health and fitness as a negative state. Plateaus are seen as a holding pattern that a person can't seem to get beyond. If you think about the meaning of the word plateau, it's really about a relatively stable period or level. How you perceive a plateau, just like how you perceive any situation, will determine if it becomes stressful for you or not.

Since we hear about plateaus mostly when it comes to

weight loss, I would venture to guess that this fear about plateaus has been created to entice you to buy more products. The reality is that plateaus mean nothing more than a temporary stable period. When it comes to weight loss, if you are losing anywhere from 20–100 pounds, your body may have a period where it stalls for a bit as you begin to release weight. If you're focused only on the numbers, you may be excited when they drop and then feel like a failure if they stall.

Instead, I encourage you to forget about the numbers and forget about plateaus. In chapter 9, where we covered Principle #5: Take Action, I addressed the idea of expecting results too quickly. Sometimes our bodies know best and we have to give them time to adjust to our new health and fitness routines.

Have you ever exercised really hard for two weeks and noticed that you looked exactly the same? That can really defeat your motivation to exercise, if all you are looking for is immediate physical changes. Now, what if instead, you tuned into how you felt? What if you noticed that you felt really good, you felt like your blood was moving and as if you had more energy when you woke up in the morning? *Rather than focusing only on numbers, take an inventory of how you feel.* That's how you recognize that success comes in many forms and you may be missing some important cues if you only look at numbers.

Here are some tips for responding to plateaus:

- TAKE AN INVENTORY OF HOW YOU FEEL. Tune into your body and your moods. Notice all of the benefits you are experiencing from inside, rather than simply focusing on the outside.

- FOCUS ON BUILDING GOOD HABITS. Recognize that a plateau is simply a stable period and trust that this is a time when you can focus on creating or maintaining good health habits. If your goal is only about losing 50 pounds, you may miss the opportunity to focus on the feeling of creating a habit that supports your well-being for a lifetime. Trust that your healthy habits will allow you to reach your goals. In this way, you can lose weight without having to stress about it.

- ACCEPT THAT SOMETIMES, THERE ARE BUMPS IN THE ROAD... AND ADJUST. Sometimes if you have a health challenge, you might have a recurrence. This has happened with me. Remember in chapter 7, when I had razor burn that went away when I eliminated dairy and then came back when I ate dairy again? This kind of recurrence can bring about the same feelings as hitting a plateau. However, when you are focused on optimal health, the goal is living the best that you can for as long as you can. When you embrace that, you can accept those bumps in the road and take action to adjust your habits.

- LOOK AT THE BIG PICTURE. On the way to reaching your health goals, you may experience slip-ups, plateaus or other challenges. Instead of getting stuck in the details along the way, what if you focused on the big picture? I'll share an example about investing in the stock market. Some people watch the stock market everyday and stress about the big ups and downs. Day traders will even take action based on those daily rises and falls, constantly moving money in and out of certain stocks. However, experts say that moving money based on these ups and downs is actually detrimental to long-term returns. In fact, it is the people who focus on the long-term picture (or the big picture) that do the best. Reacting based on market ups and downs tends to bring about the worst results.

It's the same with your health. If you focus on the little ups and downs along the way, you may miss the incredible gains you'd make over the course of a year or two years. So it's only in the moment that you're feeling down. If we can focus on the big picture — the long-term — through your entire life, you're always going to come out on top.

OVERCOME INFORMATION OVERLOAD

Another area that causes stress in our lives is information overload. We've all been there, right? How can you not these days in our information society? First of all, it's important to trust yourself. If you take the *High Raw* approach, the five principles will empower you to be your own best health advocate. Trust that you have the information you need in each moment and that you are doing your best with what you know.

Next, if you are feeling like you are overwhelmed by all the information and not sure what to do, go back and re-read chapter 9, which covers Principle #5: Take Action. Chapter 9 addresses the idea of taking everything one step at a time. Remember, stress causes a hormone reaction that is detrimental to your health. Your health and well-being will benefit more from taking things one step at a time, at your own pace, than trying to reach all of your goals overnight.

I recently re-read *The pH Miracle*, by Robert O. Young and Shelly Redford Young. I was definitely interested in alkalizing my body, because my minerals had been low. The pH Miracle has so many good suggestions that it can be easy to get overwhelmed with where to start and how much to take on. After I finished the book, I went online and ordered three products that I thought would be effective for my own health situation. I didn't do ALL of the things or take ALL of the products he recommended. After taking those three products, I felt like I had addressed what I needed to for my health and I knew I could move on. You see, I didn't have to do everything in the book because I used *High Raw* Principle #3: Know Your Body. I trusted the results of a test I had gotten done and I trusted what I knew as my own best health advocate. That allowed me to choose a small piece of what The pH Miracle suggested and move on from there.

I did the same thing when I was dealing with Lyme issues. I read *Healing Lyme: Natural Healing And Prevention of Lyme Borreliosis And Its Coinfections* by Stephen Harrod Buhner. There's a lot of information in the book, so I just chose some basic principles and took action. As I mastered those principles, I kept reading and adding new ones. This eliminated the overwhelm because instead of trying to tackle the 50 recommendations in the book, I chose a place to start and practiced that until I was ready for the next step.

Here's the key: start with one thing. Just do it. Take action on it. Get it done, then move on to the next step. When you can grasp this, you've got it made. Add to this the unshakable confidence that you know you'll achieve your goals and you can relax and enjoy the process of creating optimal health!

As they say, attitude is everything — and that's true when it comes to achieving your health goals too. When I was dealing with Candida, I said, "I know I'm going to get over this!" When I was dealing with Lyme, I told myself the same thing. I didn't want sympathy from anyone, what I DID want was to get better. And that's the attitude that I really recommend you have, because it's going to really work for you. Know that it's just going to happen. Instead of saying, "I'm going to fight it," say, "Let's go! I'm going to rock and roll. I'm going to transform my health. I'm going to figure out what's going on here, and I'm going to take care of it. And if I need to, I'm going to find people to help me get there."

Trust your intuition, but be safe too. Remember *High Raw* Principle #3: Know Your Body. Get tested. Figure out what's going on and how to know when it's resolved.

MONEY CONCERNS — CAN YOU AFFORD GOOD HEALTH?

When it comes to investing in your health, I'm going to take a tough love approach because there's nothing more important than your health. When you receive my newsletter, I have a quote at the bottom that says: "Most people work hard and spend their health trying to achieve wealth. Then they retire and spend their wealth trying to get back their health."

The thing is, what do you have if you lose your health? I think health is the most important thing, which is why *High Raw* Principle #2 is Make Health Your TOP Priority. When you make your health your top priority, nothing gets in the way, even money. In my own life, I've seen this principle in action. There were times I did not have $100 for a test that I knew I needed, but I made it happen because I knew that the test would help me achieve my health goals.

When someone comes to me and says, "I know I need this supplement, but I can't afford it because it's $20," I ask: "Do you have cable television? Do you need that? What else do you have that you don't really need that's less important than your health?"

The reality is a lot of things are less than important than your health. I would almost go out on a limb and say almost everything is less important than your health...including your cable TV and your cell phone. So many people pay big monthly bills for these items and yet, don't want to invest in their health. It's up to you to decide what's more important to you.

I've gotten emails from people who make $5,000 a year and they still eat organic foods. They've figured it out. They've found a way because they've prioritized their health. So you can find a way to afford organic food, supplements, tests or whatever you need to be healthy or reach optimal health. When you recognize that it's all about your priorities, you'll find a way to make it work.

So, how can you afford to do this? Well, what you can do is start somewhere. What I've always found is that if I stretch my comfort level when it comes to finances, over time there's always enough. For example, when my wife, Annmarie, and I wanted to buy a water filter, we could only afford a $100 water filter. We started there and then upgraded to a $300 water filter. Next time we buy a house we might buy a whole-house filter. What's important is that we started somewhere and built to a better filter from there. And each time, we focused on the fact that we had the best water we could have at that time. And we felt good.

Maybe you live near a spring and can get free water. In Moab, Utah, there's a spring that you can access from the road and people show up on Sundays and fill their jugs for the week. In that case, you don't even need a filter because you may have free solutions available to you.

Here are some tips for making your health more affordable:

- TAKE SMALL STEPS. If you feel you can't afford to buy organic food, start with just one food at a time and plan to add more as your budge allows. Maybe switch your regular lettuce to organic lettuce. Sometimes, just the act of taking that one step is the fuel for finding other solutions. Maybe you'll start gardening or sprouting. Maybe you'll find that you eat less organic food because it is so mineral rich. Perhaps an opportunity for additional work comes your way, so you can earn more money. In any case, taking a small step may lead to bigger steps AND it will certainly empower you to feel you are taking charge of your health.

- CULTIVATE A BELIEF IN ABUNDANCE. When you start from an attitude of "I can do this, I'll make it happen," everything starts to change. If you're not sure, just say that and feel what it would be like to believe it. Now say, "I can't do it, I can't afford it," and see how that makes you feel. When you believe in yourself and in abundance, it always shows up. That may sound silly — and it certainly does not mean going beyond your means — but cultivating a belief in abundance can truly bring about amazing results. Practice this for yourself and see what happens.

- FIND FREE ALTERNATIVES. If you are creative and open-minded, you may be able to reduce your costs by seeking free alternatives. One example is bartering (trading) with health experts for their services. You may have a skill — say you're a massage therapist — you can trade your skill for theirs. So you provide a free massage and they provide a free consultation. Be willing to talk to people and negotiate a trade that works for both of you. People do this all the time, especially in small businesses. You may be able to trade for products as well, so be open-minded and don't be afraid to ask! Whether you live near a fresh spring or have some space to start a garden, you may be able to lower your costs significantly. Some well known people in the raw food movement actually forage for food and superfoods in fields and forests.

- **Do a "systems check."** One of the pitfalls in achieving health goals is thinking you need every supplement and every health product. For example, you may read about symptoms and protocols and think you have a health condition that requires all of the recommended supplements. What if you ran a systems check on your body instead? Planes get a systems check before they take off and we can do the same things ourselves. Write down the systems in your body and do a check on each of them. You might find out that there's only one area you want to address. This way, you can avoid all of the supplements or most of the steps in a protocol. You can zero in on what you really do need to take and start there. This is also a place where *High Raw* Principle #3: Know Your Body is incredibly helpful. The more you know, the easier it will be to run a systems check and zero in on what you truly need.

By now you are probably starting to see a theme: you can do it. When you believe you can achieve optimal health — when you have embraced *High Raw* Principle #2: Make Your Health Your TOP Priority — you can make it happen. Along the way, there may be stumbling blocks. Everyone experiences them and if you trust that they are a normal part of the process, you can practice the techniques in this chapter and keep moving forward. You may even find, like I did, that you learn more about yourself along the way, that challenges exist only to make us stronger. And in your case, when you look at the big picture and stick to your goals, they exist to make you even healthier.

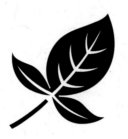

CHAPTER 14

FOOD, SUPERFOODS AND SWEETENERS

Is diet the most important aspect of achieving optimal health? After reading chapter 12, you can see that I believe optimal health is an outcome not of food alone, but of creating a healthy lifestyle. When you take a *High Raw* approach, you are eating mostly raw, ripe, organic vegetables, fruits, nuts and seeds — but that's not all. The *High Raw* lifestyle incorporates breath, plenty of pure water and exercise. Over time, you are adding all of these into your life. A healthy *High Raw* lifestyle would recognize the importance of living your passion, reducing stress and having fun.

In today's terms, many diets are sold as magic pills — quick fixes for whatever ails you. In reality, the healthiest people have had healthy lifestyles of which diet was only one part. Think of this like the

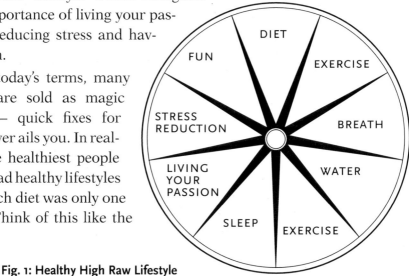

Fig. 1: Healthy High Raw Lifestyle

If you want some more in-depth information about the raw food diet from the experts in the fields of nutrition and diet, please take a look at "The Rawkathon" which is a full set of informative videos and audios to help you put these principles into your daily life! www.Rawkathon.com

spokes on a wheel. Each spoke is important for the proper functioning of the wheel because the wheel will not turn on one or two spokes alone.

Okinawa, a collection of islands south of Japan, is inhabited by some of the healthiest people alive. *The Okinawa Program: How the World's Longest-Lived People Achieve Everlasting Health — And How You Can Too*, by Dr. Bradley J. Willcox, Dr. D. Craig Willcox and Dr. Makoto Suzuki, was a best- selling book that found Okinawans to have the world's longest disability-free lives.

Their secret was all about their lifestyle — including a healthy diet that is 86% plant-based and a focus on meditation, exercise, low stress and spirituality. So recognizing that food is only one aspect of lifestyle, let's talk about food from a *High Raw* perspective.

EATING FOR OPTIMAL HEALTH

High Raw Principle #1 is eat real food and think like a raw foodist — so does this mean that raw food the only way to achieve optimal health and beauty? Not at all — however, eating more raw foods is certainly going to help.

As I've worked with many of the top health and nutrition experts, I've noticed one thing in common: they emphasize whole foods and a largely plant-based diet, whether raw or cooked.

Here are some examples of health experts who focus on a healthy lifestyle, including variations on a plant-based diet:

- SUSAN SMITH JONES, PHD., one of America's premier health experts and author of several books about nutrition and lifestyle, is an advocate of raw foods.

- JONNY BOWDEN, author and nutrition and health expert, eats a very low carbohydrate diet consisting of fish, greens, seaweeds and a little bit of brown rice. In his early sixties, he looks much younger than his age.

- JACK LALANNE, is a 94-year old fitness and nutrition expert who continues to workout every day for 2 hours. He eats grains, fish, soy, raw vegetables and green juices; and he avoids dairy, sugar and most meat.

These health experts agree that fitness and lifestyle make a big difference when it comes to health and longevity.

Here are some guidelines for eating healthy,
the **High Raw** *way:*

- REMEMBER *HIGH RAW* PRINCIPLE #1: Eat Raw Food and Think Like a Raw Foodist.

   (1) Eat 75%–95% whole, raw fruits, vegetables, nuts and seeds.

   (2) Eat 0–20% cooked vegetables, steamed vegetables, cooked legumes and cooked grains.

   (3) Use the remaining 5% for FUN! You decide what fun means to you. Whether it means more raw food, animal protein or dessert, this is your time to play and enjoy yourself.

- CHOOSE ORGANIC, WHENEVER POSSIBLE. Higher in minerals and free of harmful pesticides, organic food is tops when it comes to nutrition.

- FIND OUT WHAT WORKS FOR YOU. When deciding how much fat, protein and carbohydrates to eat, experiment and see what works for you — otherwise, you will get caught up in the disagreements among nutrition experts about what works best. This is one of those topics where you can find completely opposite views, depending upon what you listen to or what you read.

To find out the percentage of fats, carbohydrates and protein that works for you, test it. Try it out and see what works. Keep a food diary if you need to and write down what happens as you experiment. Use the information in chapter 7 about Principle #3: Know Your Body, which gives you guidelines to see what's happening in your body.

Fats

I believe that we're not meant to eat a lot of fats. While healthy fats have many benefits, too much fat can slow your body down. Fats slow down your digestion and decrease the amount of glycogen available to your body, which in essence, means you have less available energy.

Sugar

Sugar is basically a simple carbohydrate that speeds your body up. Even if you eat too much natural sugar from fruit, your blood can become too acidic. Too much sugar can lead to mineral loss and other issues, like candida, teeth issues and mood swings.

Carbohydrates

Whole foods would include complex carbohydrates, like

quinoa, millet and amaranth. Complex carbohydrates provide energy like sugars, but they break down more slowly and do not cause the kind of blood sugar spike that simple carbohydrates do. Complex carbohydrates are also good food for your gut flora — the beneficial bacteria that helps keep your digestion and immunity strong.

Protein

The building blocks of healthy cells, tissues, muscles, hormones and enzymes, protein is very important. However, I don't believe that we need to be following a high protein diet. When you are eating whole foods, you will get plenty of protein. Whole grains, like quinoa and millet are a good source of protein and you will see many plant-based foods in this chapter (in the Superfoods section) that are protein-rich, like nuts and seeds.

THE RAW FOOD DIET AND FAT, SUGAR AND CARBOHYDRATES

For those following a raw food diet, fat is often one of the main sources of calories because it's hard to fulfill caloric needs with only raw vegetables. I'd rather see people move towards a diet that includes more carbohydrates, with less protein and fat, rather than eating a lot of fat and very little carbohydrates.

The complex carbohydrates that you get from whole grains, like cooked millet and quinoa, will give your body energy without spiking your blood sugar like too much fruit or processed food.

Millet, quinoa and amaranth are alkaline grains that are really from the seed family. If you want to eat them raw, you can sprout them and even dehydrate them. If you want to eat them cooked, you can soak or sprout them and then cook them or bake them into bread. You may find, as I have, that cooking these grains makes them easier to digest. In the debate about cooking vs. raw, those who advocate cooked foods do so because in some cases, certain nutrients and digestibility is improved with cooking. I recommend you check this out for yourself and see if you find grains easier to digest when eaten raw or cooked.

One of the main tenets in the raw food movement is that cooking foods results in a loss of enzymes. While this is true, it's important to keep in mind the big picture when it comes to your diet. Enzymes are a part of the picture and if you eat the *High Raw* way, you will be getting plenty of enzymes in your diet. At the same time, it's important to think beyond enzymes to other important aspects like: vitamins and minerals and fulfilling your energy (calorie) requirements. When you are balancing these aspects of your diet, you don't have to worry about whether you are losing some enzymes when cooking grains.

THE RAW FOOD DIET, WEIGHT LOSS AND CALORIE REQUIREMENTS

Many people say, "When I eat raw food, I lose weight like crazy." This rapid weight loss is often explained as reducing your toxic load. This may be true to some degree because toxins are stored in fat cells, however, there's another reason you may be losing too much weight: you may not be getting enough calories. Your body needs a certain amount of calories to fulfill your basal metabolic needs. It's not uncommon to consume too few calories on the raw food diet, especially one that emphasizes mostly vegetables, low fat and lower amounts of nuts and seeds.

This happened to me when I went on the raw food diet. I began to lose too much weight, so I began following Doug Graham's 80/10/10 approach and eating more fruit. The fruit helped me get more calories and I was able to gain the weight back, which was great. Unfortunately it happened at the same time that I had Lyme disease, when I was taking an antibiotic. Antibiotics kill bad bacteria, but they also kill good bacteria, so I developed candida (a systemic yeast infection). So you can see what happens when you start to change things in your diet. The important thing to remember is what works for you — and that may change depending upon your health circumstances at the time. In the meantime, getting enough calories is important for feeling your best and maintaining your weight.

Many people following the raw food diet may end up eating too much sugar from fruit to meet their calorie needs. Even if you don't have a Lyme or candida issue, I still think too much fruit can be problematic because it can create an acidic blood condition, which can contribute to illness and disease. Adding cooked grains is a really good solution for boosting your calories so that you don't need to consume an overabundance of fat or fruit sugar.

While I believe healthy fats and fruit is important, you can end up eating too much of both of these foods on a 100% raw food diet simply to meet your calorie needs. Instead, you could add calories and density to your food by adding some things that are slightly cooked, like steamed vegetables and cooked grains.

If you are losing too much weight, think about how you can incorporate more calories into your diet. Go online and find a little calorie calculator — they're everywhere. Take a look at what your basic metabolic rate would be and how many calories you burn.

Now I'm not tied to calories as the way to measure how much food you should be eating or not, or anything like that. I simply want to emphasize that your body does have an energy requirement. You do require energy. In order for your system to really function optimally, you need to get the energy that your system requires. This is how you allow your body to do the amazing things that human bodies do — like healing itself. If you're giving your body the energy it needs, it will be much more willing to stay healthy and youthful.

SUPERFOODS

Superfoods are foods that are prized for their high concentration of nutrients. We hear a lot about them in health and nutrition, but what's the real deal on superfoods? If you are following *High Raw* Principle #1 and eating an abundance of whole, raw, ripe plant foods, you will be getting plenty of nutrients.

It is not necessary to focus your whole diet on superfoods. Some superfoods may seem exotic and expensive, yet there are many easy-to-find and affordable options. I am going to cover some of my favorite superfoods and concentrate on those that are readily available and make excellent additions to a regular diet.

Green vegetables and green juices

Land vegetables are nature's best superfood. Readily available in supermarkets, farmer's markets, health food stores or your own backyard, they are rich in vitamins, minerals and antioxidants. Kale, collards, romaine lettuce, parsley, arugula, spinach, mustard greens and escarole are just some examples of healthy greens. I have found green juices to be one of the best ways to get a lot of greens into your diet that also hydrate and energize your body. Green juices are one of my staple superfoods.

Sea vegetables

Also called seaweed, are grown in an environment full on minerals that your body needs for optimal health — the ocean. Ocean water has up to 92 minerals can be absorbed by the plants growing in the sea. This makes sea vegetables one of the most nutrient dense foods on the planet. Sea vegetables, when compared to land vegetables, are one of the best vegetable sources of calcium, which is fantastic for muscle and bone development, strength and growth.

Don't worry if the idea of eating seaweed grosses you out. Your health food store will have different seaweed granules that you can use as a salt substitute and you'll never know the difference. Nori, dulce, and kelp are three of the most readily available sea vegetables.

Pumpkin Seeds

The raw pumpkin seed is a feel-good food because it's a great source of tryptophan, the amino acid precursor to serotonin (the feel good hormone). Pumpkin seeds also are excellent sources of protein, fat and other essential minerals, like magnesium. You can find this super-seed right in your backyard if you live in the Northeastern US! Add them to salads as an extra garnish, use them for snacking or mix them in with other superfoods.

Pumpkin seeds can promote weight loss along with other seeds, like hemp seed, flax seed and raw sunflower seeds.

Hemp Seeds

Hemp seeds are considered to be one of the most nutritious food sources on the planet. They contain vitamin E, Omega-3 oils, GLA, and have an extremely high composition of protein. This protein is called edistin, which can be used by the body in its raw state, unlike soybeans, which have to be cooked or sprouted.

The hemp seed is 33% protein by volume! It is a fantastic source of protein for the athlete who doesn't want to — or can't — stomach pounds and pounds of turkey and chicken. Hemp seeds have essential fatty acids (EFAs), like omega-3's and omega-6s, which are important for optimal health. Hemp also contains three times the vitamin E contained in flax seeds. You can add hemp seeds to almost anything! A salad, a desert, your breakfast... they have a light nutty flavor, almost like a sunflower seed.

Maca

Maca is a Peruvian root powder that is used to increase strength and vitality. It has more mineral content than potatoes and carrots — containing iron, magnesium, calcium, potassium, and iodine. The Peruvians and many others claim, maca can help fight depression, help with anemia and improve overall memory and vitality. This powerful food is also a libido stimulant!

Maca powder is best taken mixed with warm water in a tea. It has a strong taste and this can be softened with goji berries or honey.

Cacao

I get a lot of questions about cacao because everyone wants to know about raw chocolate. Cacao is rich in magnesium and also a good source of arginine, tryptophan and antioxidants. For me personally, raw chocolate and I do not get along. I used to be a fan of cacao, eating it everyday in powdered form and nibs.

After some testing, I confirmed the symptoms I was having when eating cacao everyday. I ended up with adrenal stress, eczema, low minerals and acidic pH, which affected my kidneys. After doing the two-week experiments that I recommend in chapter 7, I found that it was the cacao causing these symptoms. When I eliminated the cacao, the symptoms

I had, like dark urine and eczema, went away.

Cacao is a stimulant because it contains theobromine, a chemical related to caffeine. Most people who eat cacao will tell you that it gives them a little boost, much like caffeine. For me, eating the quantity of cacao I did every day was not good. I encourage you to experiment and make your own decision about cacao. You may find, like I did, that it makes a better occasional treat than an everyday staple.

There are many other superfoods out there to learn about and experiment with. When it comes to superfoods or any food, it's important to decide what works for you because that's what *High Raw* is all about.

SWEETENERS

Sugar consumption has continued to rise over the past fifty years and after reading chapter 13, you are aware that I think the less sugar we eat, the better. This includes natural sugars found in fruit and other sweeteners.

However, the sweet taste is a natural part of any diet. In Ayurvedic medicine, sweet is just one of six tastes that also include sour, bitter, pungent and astringent. As you follow *High Raw* Principle #1, you will be eating more whole, ripe, raw plant-based foods. As your body gets the nutrients it needs, you may find that you crave sweets less and less. You may wonder why you ever needed to add sugar and sweeteners in the first place.

But what is the best sweetener to use if you find you want to satisfy your sweet tooth? I believe that raw honey is the best sweetener because it is the most natural.

Here is an overview of some of the most popular sweeteners:

Raw Honey

When it comes to raw honey, I'm not talking about the honey in the little bear. I'm talking real, unprocessed, raw honey. Raw honey contains enzymes, phytonutrients, resins and propolis, which is bee glue. This unique combination of properties makes it versatile not only as a food, but as an anti-bacterial agent.

As a food, raw honey can raise antioxidant levels in the body, restore muscle glycogen after a workout and help lower cholesterol and the risk of certain cancers. As a topical substance, it can decrease infection and work just as well as alcohol solutions. Used as a sweetener, you can put some in your teas or your water, or just have a small spoonful for a quick pick me up. If you want the full benefits of raw honey, just be sure not to heat it to a high temperature. Heat will destroy many of its best qualities.

Agave

There's a debate about whether agave is a good sweetener or not. Agave is a processed sweetener. They take the agave syrup, they distill it down to a semi-sweetness attached to the actual fiber molecule and then they add an enzyme to separate the sugar from it. What's separated is the agave nectar. People will argue that agave is fairly natural because of the added enzymes, but you can't compare this to the natural process of bees making raw honey. There's nothing in nature that takes the agave liquid, boils it down (often at temperatures exceeding 140 degrees F), distills it and then throws an enzyme on it to make it a sugar.

Maple Syrup

Maple syrup is processed as well, although perhaps a bit less than agave. Maple sap, once collected from trees, is not very sweet. Maple syrup gets its sweetness after being boiled down to a more concentrated state.

Yacon Syrup

Raw yacon syrup is heated to 104 degrees F, so while it is more processed than honey, it is considered raw. Yacon syrup is becoming a popular sweetener for raw foodists.

Stevia

Stevia, another processed sweetener, is an herb that is 300 times sweeter than sugar. You only need a tiny pinch of stevia to get a sweet taste — using too much results in a bitter aftertaste. Stevia is being used by a lot of corporations who want to use natural sweeteners instead of artificial sweeteners. For this reason, you'll find more and more products using stevia, which I don't think is necessarily a good thing. With the abundance of sweet foods in the standard American diet, we don't know the long-term effects of eating a lot of stevia. If you were just putting a little pinch in a few things here and there, that's one thing, but using stevia in everything from sodas to tea, bread and cookies and consumed in high amounts is questionable.

Take a look at what you are eating and see how often you feel a desire for sweet foods. Notice if there are sweeteners being added to foods that don't even need it — like dressing, for example. Experiment with leaving the sweetener out or a recipe completely or cutting it in half. You may not even miss it. And if you continue to find yourself craving sugar or sweeteners, read the section on eliminating cravings in chapter 13. There are many excellent techniques that can help you reduce or eliminate the pull you feel toward sugar and sweeteners.

A POWERFUL EXERCISE TO MOVE TOWARD A HEALTHIER DIET: THE PROCESS OF ADDING

So you're ready to eat healthier, but maybe you don't like the thought of taking things out of your diet. This is not an uncommon feeling because most of the time, when something is taken away, we want it back. If it doesn't feel good to eliminate things from your diet, here's a really powerful process that can help you transition into a healthier diet without a feeling of deprivation. I learned this process from raw food expert, David Wolfe.

The key is, instead of eliminating things from your diet, add healthy food into your current diet. While this example is a bit extreme, it illustrates the point: let's say pizza is your favorite food and you eat it every day. If I told you to eliminate pizza and start eating salad instead, you'd probably protest. Perhaps you'd be able to do it for a short period of time, maybe two weeks, but you'd probably be looking at the calendar and waiting to add your pizza back. Now you're focused on what you can't have, instead of what you can have.

Instead, how about adding something healthy to what you are already eating? To do this, start using *High Raw* Principle #1: Eat Real Food and Think Like a Raw Foodist. With this mindset, you start where you are and build on what you are doing already. Let's say you have pizza for breakfast, sticking to your usual routine. At lunch, you ask yourself, "What can I add to this pizza to make it healthier?" Perhaps you add some romaine lettuce – just drop it right on top of your pizza. At dinner time, you ask again, "What can I add to this pizza to make it healthier?" Now you are building on what you did at lunch, so maybe you add some lettuce and some slices of onion.

With each meal, you are adding more healthy ingredients to your pizza. Eventually, you may replace half of your pizza with a salad. Over time, your body will start to cleanse and you will eliminate the pizza at a pace that works for you. Your body will support you by developing a taste for healthier foods.

With each meal, ask yourself, "How can I make this healthier?" In this way, instead of focusing on eliminating food, you are focusing on continuous improvement. I am not suggesting, however, that there is some pinnacle that is the absolute healthiest way to eat. And I am certainly not suggesting that we aim for subsisting on breath and water alone. What I am suggesting is that you think of the way you eat as a growing process. If you relax and trust that you are always growing and progressing, you don't have to stress out about whether you are eating "the perfect diet."

Keep in mind that this process of adding will likely take a little bit of time. It's OK to take this at your own pace — you are creating healthy habits for a lifetime. Sometimes, people ask me, "Kevin, how do you eat so healthy?" and my response is that it's been years in the making. I didn't start out eating healthy – remember, I was into Twinkies, pizza and beer at one time. I like to think of myself as a work in progress and I think we all are to some degree. If you trust where you are, rather than comparing yourself to another person or a standard that feels difficult to attain, it takes the fun out of this whole journey toward optimal health. Take your time and trust that you will keep moving forward from where you are.

HEALTH AND BEAUTY FROM THE INSIDE OUT

When you embrace the *High Raw* lifestyle, you will be eating more whole foods, including ripe, raw vegetables and fruits. You may find that this one habit alone will be a major beauty secret that will bring you a youthful glow and plenty of energy. But remember that we are talking about creating a lifestyle that supports feeling your best – and that food is only one part of the picture. Breath, water, exercise, plenty of sleep, reduced stress and doing what you love — having fun — is the real beauty secret.

As you take these steps at your own pace, don't be surprised if you start to throw away those beauty creams and cosmetics you once thought you needed to look great. A *High Raw* lifestyle promotes health and beauty from the inside out. You unlock your body's potential to heal and glow with youthful energy. Good health is simply the best way to look and feel your best.

CHAPTER 15

SUPPLEMENTS

One of the most common questions I get on my blog at www. RenegadeHealth.com is "What supplements should I take?" In this chapter, I will share my views on the best supplements to take and more importantly, my philosophy on supplements as a whole.

First of all, *High Raw* Principle #3: Know Your Body — is key when it comes to which supplements are best for you. Anyone can give you a list of the best supplements, but each person is different. When you get tested to find out what your specific needs are, you will get more for your money. Chapter 7 outlines several options for tests to help you determine nutrient deficiencies. Maybe you'll find out you don't need supplements at all – or perhaps you'll only need one or two. You'll save a lot of time and money when you have that information.

When you are following a healthy *High Raw* lifestyle, you will likely be getting most of the nutrients you need from food, so a lot of supplements may not be necessary. However, there are certain supplements that I recommend because they offer a kind of "nutritional back up plan," that I often think of as "insurance" for my best health. In this chapter,

I'm going to outline my favorite supplements that are great additions to any health routine.

An important guideline to keep in mind is to look for supplements that are made from whole foods or whole food extracts. Unless you have a severe deficiency, taking supplements made from whole foods or whole food extracts are ideal for regular use.

You may not realize that all supplements are really only sourced from five or six labs around the country. This means that when you choose high quality supplements, there's not that much variation between product A and product B. But not all supplements are created equally. The low quality supplements that you find for bargain basement prices in the local vitamin store are bottom of the barrel when it comes to quality.

I've heard horror stories about fish oils. Some fish oils are actually rancid by the time it gets made into capsules. You may not even know it when you are taking them, so looking at how a product is made can also help you choose the best quality product. Know your supplement producer — call them up and ask them how their products are produced.

Here are some excellent supplements for a regular health regimen:

Green Powder

Green powders are an incredible foundation for your regular health routine. And if you are looking for an easy way to boost your health, adding green powder is the way to go.

Green powders provide vitamins, minerals and phytonutrients that you may not get in your regular diet. With a high quality green powder, you only need a small daily amount to cover all your bases when combined with a healthy diet. While a green powder alone is a great way to start a healthy eating program, you'll still want to focus on a diet full of whole, ripe, raw greens. In other words, the green drink does not make up for a diet lacking in vegetables, but it does give you a good range of nutrients to help you feel your best.

Here's what to look for when choosing a high quality green powder:

- Organic or wildcrafted ingredients
- Seaweeds, like kelp, nori or dulse
- Thyroid support, like iodine.
- A full spectrum of different plants, like kale, spinach, nettles, horsetail, parsley; and grasses, like wheat grass and barley grass.
- Algae, like spirulina and chlorella
- Enzymes
- Probiotics

As you can see, green powders have a wide variety of nutrients. While the taste may take some getting used to, some of them taste better than others. Two exceptional green powders are: Vitamineral Green from HealthForce and Revitaphi from Elements for Life. You can mix green powder with water or put it in a smoothie. Adding green powder to a smoothie with banana, some water and coconut water makes a delicious mineral-rich drink.

Probiotics

Probiotics are the healthy bacteria and yeast that help boost your immunity and aid your digestion. We all have a mix of good and bad bacteria and yeast in our intestines. It's important to keep the balance right, so that you feel your best.

Anyone who has experienced chronic stress, consumed a diet full of processed foods, taken antibiotics or consumed anything that kills bacteria (like, chlorine in water), may have an imbalance of good and bad bacteria and yeast. An imbalance means you may have too many of the "bad guys," which can set the stage for illness.

You can eat food that promotes probiotics in your gut, like fermented foods (cultured vegetables, miso and tempeh) and "prebiotics." Prebiotics are food for probiotics and include foods like onions, raw apple cider vinegar, grains, fruit and certain herbs, like chicory root.

When it comes to taking probiotics, look at your lifestyle. If you are under a lot of stress or taking antibiotics, you may want to take extra probiotics to help keep the "good guys" in balance and then cut back to the regular amount you were taking.

If you are having digestive problems — and so many people do today — probiotics can help improve your digestion. If you're not digesting your food properly, you are not assimilating all of the nutrients from your food. When your flora (bacteria and yeast) are in balance, the good guys actually help you digest and assimilate your food. They even help create vitamins, like B vitamins and vitamin K.

There are many great probiotic supplements out there. My favorite is Jon Barron's products, Baseline Nutritionals Probiotics.

Enzymes

Enzymes are proteins that are involved in digestion and every chemical reaction in your body. According to food enzyme researcher, Dr. Edward Howell, "Without enzymes, no activity at all would take place. Neither vitamins, minerals, or hormones can do any work — without enzymes."[1] In fact, many health experts believe that health and longevity is directly related to your body's supply of enzymes.

Since enzymes are used up for digestion and other metabolic functions and since we lose enzymes as we age, taking enzyme supplements can help your body in a variety of ways.

The two types of enzyme supplements are:

- DIGESTIVE ENZYMES: Digestive enzymes are specifically formulated to help you digest your food. Different types of enzymes help break down carbohydrates, fats and proteins. Many people today experience digestive problems, like gas, bloating and fatigue after eating meals. Taking digestive enzymes can relieve these symptoms by helping your body fully digest and assimilate your food. I like Baseline Nutritionals Digestive Enzymes.

- SYSTEMIC ENZYMES: Systemic enzymes are taken on an empty stomach — not for digestion — but for the rest of your metabolic processes. Think of systemic enzymes like a janitor, sweeping everything out of your system to clean and detoxify your internal environment. Systemic enzymes can help boost immunity and reduce conditions like acidity, joint pain, inflammation and gout. Some really high quality systemic enzymes are Wobenzyme (not plant-based) and Dr. Fred Bisci's Therapeutic Enzymes (plant-based).

With today's stressful lifestyles, I think everyone can benefit from taking both digestive and systemic enzymes, particularly if you're having digestive issues, even if you are eating healthy. Certainly, the more raw foods you eat, the more enzymes you will have in your food, which definitely helps. But if you experience symptoms of low energy, low immunity or poor digestion, you may find that digestive and systemic enzymes can give your health a boost.

Some Signs of Vitamin B12 Deficiency Are:[3]

- Irritability
- Apathy
- Sleepiness
- Paranoia
- Personality changes
- Depression, including postpartum depression
- Memory loss
- Dementia
- Clumsiness (stiff arms or legs)
- Symptoms that appear to be Parkinson's, Alzheimer's or MS
- Incontinence
- Vision changes or optic nerve damage
- Heart palpitations, heart attack or congestive heart failure
- Shortness of breath
- Chronic fatigue or general weakness
- Poor digestion (bloated or full feeling after small or normal sized meals)
- Constipation or diarrhea
- Osteoporosis
- Vitamin D

Vitamin B12

Vitamin B12 is a very important supplement, particularly if you are following the *High Raw* lifestyle or you are a vegetarian or raw foodist. B12 is a water-soluble vitamin that cannot be stored in your body. This means you need to have adequate intake of vitamin B12 each day. B12 is found in foods like meat, poultry, eggs, fish, grains, dairy and some algae. However, experts are saying that the B12 in meat, poultry and fish is the most readily absorbed, while eggs and plant-based sources have properties that make it more difficult to absorb.

Unfortunately, even if you take a B12 vitamin or eat meat, you may not be absorbing the vitamin B12. This is because the process of breaking down vitamin B12 in your body is very complex. First, many people lack adequate hydrochloric acid (stomach acid), which means they don't have enough of the enzyme pepsin to break down vitamin B12 in the stomach. Next, many people are missing "intrinsic factor," a protein produced in your stomach that helps break down B12 in your intestines. In fact, with each step in your digestive process, there are complications that make vitamin B12 tricky to digest and assimilate.[2]

In chapter 7, you learned about the urinary MMA test for B12 deficiency and I highly recommend everyone get tested. Vitamin B12 deficiency can cause a wide variety of symptoms from irritability and depression to memory loss and chronic fatigue. While vitamin B12 deficiency is easily corrected if caught early, it can cause permanent damage if it goes untreated for too long. Since symptoms can mimic other health issues, vitamin B12 deficiency can go undiagnosed until it's too late. For this reason, it's important to get tested and know your B12 levels.

Typically, treatment for B12 deficiency would include a series of B12 shots that you can get from your health practitioner. It's typically very inexpensive. Or your health practitioner can teach you how to self-administer the shots. Some people will have to take them monthly for life. If your B12 levels are good and you only need a regular supplement, many people do well with a vitamin B12 lozenge or vitamin B12 spray. The good news is that high quality vitamin B12 is very inexpensive — the one I use is $12 for a monthly supply.

When it comes to which vitamin B12 to choose, make sure that you get methylcobalamin or hydroxycobolamin. Methylcobalamin is a much more easily absorbed version of B12, so that's what I recommend you look for. You'll know a cheap vitamin if you look at it and it says cyanocobalamin.

Symptoms of Vitamin D Deficiency:[5]

- Depression and mood swings

- Low immunity

- Sleep irregularities

- Renal problems

- Intestinal issues, like IBS or Chrohn's disease

- Fatigue or low energy

- Weak bones

Vitamin D

I recommend everyone get tested for vitamin D levels. Vitamin D is the "free vitamin" because you can get it from the sunshine. However, vitamin D deficiency is more prevalent than you may think, affecting up to 40% of Americans.[4]

When I got tested for vitamin D, I was surprised that my own levels were low, since I spend a good amount of time in the sun. Since vitamin D deficiency is linked to cancer, depression and intestinal problems, among other health issues, I highly recommend getting tested to see how your vitamin D levels are. You may want to get tested in the winter as well, if you live in a cold climate where you'd have less sun exposure. With plenty of time in the sunshine, you may not need to take vitamin D at all. Testing for vitamin D levels will help you know for sure. Chapter 7 has more information on vitamin D testing.

One thing to keep in mind is that vitamin D3, the form that your body uses, is not available from a plant-based source. If you're a really strict vegan, you might have a moral issue with this, but remember *High Raw* Principle #2: Make Your Health Your Top Priority. Your health is of the utmost importance, so you may want to consider what your body needs most of all. The good news is that you can get vitamin D3 sourced from lanolin or sheep's wool. While lanolin is an animal product, it's not a part of the huge, destructive conglomerate business that is destroying life for food. What happens is the sheep releases vitamin D2 and then the sun converts it to vitamin D3.

There are many good brands of vitamin D. I use Bio-D Mulsion Forte by Biotics Research, which provides vitamin D3 in an emulsified form. Since vitamin D is a fat-soluble vitamin, this helps with the bioavailablity. Work with a practitioner to determine how to supplement with vitamin D because you can overdo it. Your health practitioner can recommend how much you should take, particularly if you have some sort of deficiency and need to rebuild your vitamin D levels.

While there are many other excellent supplements, my goal is to highlight some of the key products to create a baseline of good health. Green powders, probiotics and enzymes are in my opinion, a kind of insurance for optimal health. Vitamins B12 and D are also critical, but just like with any other supplement you are considering, I highly recommend you get tested so that you can tailor your supplements to the needs of your body.

From time to time, you may also be looking for natural solutions for a specific health situation. The questions I get most often are about natural supplements to boost immunity, decrease inflammation, detoxify your body and fight viruses.

Here are some great herbs for your immune system:

Olive Leaf Extract
The olive leaf herb has been used since ancient Egyptian times for its medicinal properties. Research has shown that fresh olive leaf extract is higher in antioxidants that extra virgin olive oil, gogi berries, noni juice and vitamin C.[6] Most recently, due to olive leaf extracts powerful anti-viral properties, it has been getting attention as a possible avian flu remedy.

If you are experiencing a viral infection, like the flu, Epstein Barr or Lyme disease, you might consider taking olive leaf extract in the form of a tincture. Work with your health practitioner though, because there are certain contraindications for taking olive leaf tincture. For example, if you are taking antibiotics, the olive leaf tincture may decrease their effectiveness.

Cat's Claw

A vine from the Amazon and South America, cat's claw has been used for its immune-stimulating properties since the Inca civilization. Cat's claw is made from the root and bark of the vine and has properties that help reduce inflammation and fight certain viruses.[7]

Cat's claw has been studied for its benefits for osteoarthritis, rheumatoid arthritis, HIV, MS, lupus and Chrohn's disease.[8]

Cilantro

Cilantro is the leaf of the plant also known as coriander (seeds). Cilantro is used to improve digestion and fight infection. It has anti-fungal, anti-bacterial and anti-inflammatory properties. Cilantro is often used as part of natural chelation therapy, which helps remove heavy metals from your body. Cilantro has been used in many ways from simply eating the herb in salads or smoothies to making tea or using the tincture.

Oregano Oil Extract

Often included in candida and parasite cleansing formulas, oregano extract has anti-fungal, anti-bacterial, anti-viral and antiseptic properties. Oregano oil extract has been used to boost immunity and settle upset stomach, treat food poising and relieve other digestive problems.

While herbal remedies have many medicinal benefits, they may also have contraindications, so make sure you know what they are before using them. Working with a health practitioner is a great way to receive guidance on herbs that will benefit your specific health goals.

LET THY HEALTHY LIFESTYLE BE THY MEDICINE

Hippocrates, the father of medicine, is well known for saying, ""Let thy food be thy medicine and thy medicine be thy food." The *High Raw* approach embraces good nutrition as one of the pillars of optimal health. And yet, as you know from reading chapter 14, a healthy lifestyle is just as important as good nutrition.

Taking supplements can be great "insurance" for health and wellness, especially when you follow *High Raw* Principle #3: Know Your Body. However, just as important is focusing on your breath, water, exercise — and all of the components that make up your healthy lifestyle.

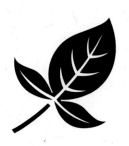

CHAPTER 16

DETOXIFICATION

BECOMING CHEMICAL FREE

Toxins are everywhere...in the air, water, food and many of the products we use. We literally cannot escape toxins, so being 100% toxin free is not realistic. Instead, when your goal is optimal health, you go a long way toward reducing exposure to toxins. The good news is that your body is designed to detoxify and when you follow the *High Raw* lifestyle, you will be reducing exposure to chemicals over time.

The idea is not to worry about toxins you can't control, but to reduce your exposure to toxic chemicals that you CAN control. Examples of toxic exposure you can control are: the food you eat, the personal care and beauty products you use, the fabrics in your clothing and furniture and the cleaning products you use in your home.

From organic foods to chemical-free cleaning and beauty products, there are many toxin-free options that put you in charge of your best health. Your *High Raw* lifestyle will also help boost your immunity, so that your body's organs of detoxification remain strong.

Your body's major organs of detoxification are:

- Liver
- Lungs
- Intestines
- Kidneys
- Skin

If you expose your body to too many toxins, over time, your detoxification pathways can get clogged. Some examples of clogged detoxification pathways are: constipation, difficulty digesting fats or not sweating very much when you exercise. This overburden of toxins can create an acidic condition in your blood, which sets the stage for illness and disease.

ACIDITY

In *The pH Miracle: Balance Your Diet, Reclaim Your Health* authors Dr. Robert O. Young and Shelley Redford Young explain that the pH of your blood is supposed to be slightly alkaline. However, too many people have acidic blood because of lifestyle habits like poor diet, lack of hydration, stress and exposure to toxins. According to the authors, it is this acidic blood that leads to all major diseases we know of today.

The pH Miracle outlines a strategy to get your blood back to its desired alkaline state through an diet that consists of 80% alkaline-forming foods, like green vegetables. When you follow the *High Raw* lifestyle, you will be consuming more alkaline-forming foods. Keep in mind that acidic blood strips your body of minerals, so when you eat a mineral rich diet, you can begin to correct deficiencies you may be experiencing.

Combining good nutrition with lifestyle habits — like exercise, drinking pure water and green juices, taking deep breaths and reducing stress — can help your blood come to a more alkaline state.

In addition, some of the supplements I covered in chapter 15 are very valuable for bringing your blood back to a more alkaline state. Green powder drinks, probiotics and digestive and systemic enzymes are excellent supplements for alkalizing your blood. If you get tested and find you have mineral deficiencies, you may want to supplement with minerals as well, until you get your body back into balance. Some examples are colloidal minerals and Quinton.

The Youngs further suggest that the systemic yeast (fungal) infection, candida, is also a culprit of today's poor health. The good news is, as you alkalize your blood, you are creating a condition that is inhospitable for bacterial and fungal infections, like candida.

CANDIDA

Candida is a microorganism that is part of the typical gut flora in everyone's body. However, with poor diet and lifestyle habits, an imbalance in gut flora can occur and a candida overgrowth may result. This systemic yeast or fungal infection is also called Candidiasis. Symptoms are wide-ranging from digestive pain, like gas and bloating to fatigue, cravings and memory issues.

Having experienced candida myself, I have found a protocol that works for me. While this section is only intended to briefly introduce candida, I will be coming out with guidelines on how to eliminate candida. Keep in mind that as you follow the *High Raw* lifestyle, you will be putting habits in place that help keep your gut flora in balance. It's important to recognize that when you reduce toxins and start eating a healthy diet, you may feel a bit worse for a short period. This is known as "die-off" reaction.

DIE-OFF REACTION

Die-off reaction, also called Herxheimer reaction or a "healing crisis," is very common when you start to eat healthy and improve your lifestyle. Die-off is when your symptoms seem to intensify as you switch to a healthy diet and lifestyle. The reason symptoms intensify is because pathogens are dying and being released into your system so that you can eliminate them.

If you have candida, heavy metal toxicity or a serious illness, you may experience more die-off symptoms than others. Because of symptoms like die-off, it's important to pay attention to *High Raw* Principle #3: Know Your Body. Remember that your body is made to detoxify. Sometimes, symptoms you experience may be detoxification, other times die-off and still other times, you may experience symptoms because you are doing something your body does not want you to do — or perhaps your body really needs something, like more minerals.

If you are experiencing symptoms and you don't know why, read chapter 7 and consider the two-week experiments and working with a health practitioner. The more you get to know your body, the easier it will be to identify what's happening as you continue on your journey to optimal health.

One thing to note if you are experiencing die-off is the importance of keeping your detoxification pathways open. You can do this by exercising, spending time in a sauna, dry skin brushing and drinking plenty of water. If you are constipated, you might want to consider colon cleansing.

COLON CLEANSING

Colon cleansing, also called "colonics" or colon hydrotherapy, is a way to cleanse your large intestine of impacted fecal matter, pathogens and toxins. When you get a colonic, your large intestine is gently flushed with water to break up old, hardened matter from the walls of your intestine. Colonics hydrate and exercise the muscle of your colon.

Colon cleansing does more than help your colon detoxify. Once your large intestine releases toxins, your liver is freed up to release toxins and your cells can release toxins too, giving your whole body a chance to detoxify. This is why you might notice benefits from colon cleansing that surprise you, like better skin or relief from symptoms like headaches.

How often you get colonics is up to you, based on how well you know your body. A colon hydrotherapist can also help you determine the right plan for you. I recommend colon cleansing once per quarter as part of a regular cleansing routine.

You can also do internal colon cleanses with psyllium, pectin and a clay-type powder. Dr. Shulze's 5-Day Bowel Detox and Jon Barron's Colon Detoxifier are two examples. These products contain ingredients that help sweep toxins from your colon wall. When you eat a high fiber diet, which you are doing by following *High Raw*, the fiber helps to sweep toxins out of your body as well.

Colon cleansing is a good place to start in any detoxification program. Once your colon is cleansed, you may want to do a deeper cleanse, focusing on other organs of detoxification.

LIVER, GALLBLADDER AND KIDNEY FLUSHES

Liver, gallbladder and kidney flushes are good to do every once in awhile. While you don't have to be eating healthy or even eating a raw food diet during these cleanses, I highly recommend that you combine any type of cleansing with a healthy diet. Raw foods are particularly cooling and cleansing to the body and they help your liver detoxify, so raw food can be very helpful with liver and gallbladder flushes.

The liver, gallbladder and kidney flushes that I like are Dr. Shulze's 5-Day Liver Detox, which benefits your liver and gall bladder and Dr. Shulze's 5-Day Kidney Detox. These powerful products are full of organic and wildcrafted herbs that help your liver, gallbladder and kidney detoxify.

I'm not a big fan of the Epsom salts and the gallstone flushes. It's definitely not gallstones that you're expelling in those types of cleanses. Instead, you are eliminating a kind of emulsification of all the stuff you're eating as well as from the bile that's coming out. It can work, but if you do have some kind of blockage, it could be dangerous as well. While you can do these cleanses on your own, it can help to have a health practitioner or some type of guidance to answer your questions during cleanses like this.

FASTING

Many health experts recommend fasting as a way to give your digestive system a break from time to time. Depending upon what you read or who you ask, it seems that everyone has a different opinion on how to fast, how long to fast and how often to fast.

While I agree that fasting could be beneficial, this is an area where I'd recommend working with an expert. There are many things to consider when deciding whether fasting will be right for you.

I'm not a big fan of water fasting or extensive juice fasting, unless you have a real health reason for doing it and you have supervision. Some people become addicted to fasting, worrying that their bodies are full of toxins and fasting is the only way to eliminate them. This kind of thinking can be very harmful. Remember, one of the keys to the *High Raw* approach is fun. If focusing on health becomes more about worrying whether your body is full of toxins, you will no longer be having fun. In fact, you'll probably be experiencing stress, which creates an acidic condition and kills beneficial gut flora.

I do think we need to give our bodies a break from time to time. But you might think of it more like a vacation. Maybe you give your body a break from cooked foods for a week and just eat greens as a type of fast. Maybe you give your body a break from stress for a week — you might see equally good benefits. The concept of giving your body a break and refocusing on healthy habits is certainly a good one.

It's kind of like what I did with cacao. I thought it was so healthy that I went off track from the basics and started eating too much cacao. I just went into that realm of "this is the best food for me" and it turned out that it wasn't. Whereas, if I'd just focused on the Five Principles of *High Raw*, I would realize I had gone off track from the basics — fresh vegetables, nuts, fruits, seeds, maybe some grains, maybe some legumes. Once I refocused on that, I felt a lot better. And the funny thing is, it's so easy!

Being healthy does not have to be complicated. When you trust that your body is always detoxifying — that it was designed to detoxify — then you can trust that following the *High Raw* lifestyle will go a long way toward meeting your detox needs. There is a time and a place for everything, including detox. When you follow *High Raw* Principle #3 Know Your Body, you will know whether and when a detoxification program is right for you.

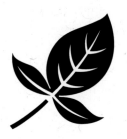

CHAPTER 17

SHARING YOUR HIGH RAW JOURNEY

SPREADING THE HIGH RAW MESSAGE

As you get into the *High Raw* lifestyle, you will probably start feeling so good that you want to share what you are doing with others. Many people ask me questions about how to share the message and I often say that I'd rather talk about religion and politics (in the same conversation!) than talk about food. Why? After reading chapter 2, you probably realize that with so much controversial information out there about food and health, it can be difficult to change people's minds about what is healthy.

What WILL change people's minds is seeing your results. When your energy skyrockets, you recover from a health condition, your skin improves, you look younger, you seem calmer or you lose weight – people start to pay attention. It is your positive results that will convince people more than any words you say.

Therefore, in order to spread the message of health — of this simple *High Raw* lifestyle — you have to live it. Become confident and comfortable with the *High Raw* lifestyle at your own pace. Become so confident in your healthy lifestyle that no one's opinion can knock you down. Feel so good about what you are doing that no matter what opinions you hear, you can say, "All I know is that I feel great and this feels right."

When you are following *High Raw* Principle #1: Eat Real Food and Think Like a Raw Foodist, the most basic principle is whole foods and plenty of raw, ripe fruits and vegetables. As people see you get results, they will be asking what you are doing. The simplest thing you can tell them is that you are focusing on a plant-based diet of whole foods and plenty of raw, ripe fruits and vegetables. What could be easier than that? This is something just about anyone could understand.

Here's what I do when I'm with my family around the holidays: when they pass me some processed food, I say to them, "Oh, I'm doing this experiment." At this point, everyone in my family is used to my experiments, so there's a bit of laughter as they ask me what it is this time. I might simply say, "I'm not eating meat." Or, "I'm eating as many raw vegetables as possible because I hear it's good for you." I have found that this tends to eliminate the need to to argue and talk about all of the angles around one type of diet or another. At this point, I might say, "Want to hear more about it?" and if they say yes, I have an invitation to share. If they say no, I will not share more about it — because I recognize they are not interested or not ready to hear more at that time. No matter what I say, that is the reality.

What I am suggesting is that instead of taking your *High Raw* message to your family or even to a community (senior citizens, school children, etc.), instead of making a point to educate them, take a step back. It is much more successful if you find out what they are interested in, what their needs are or what problems they want to solve and start from there.

For example, if you want to take the *High Raw* message to

a group of senior citizens, you might not be successful unless you can find out if they even care. Perhaps the group is more interested in how to make ends meet on a fixed income or how to save money. Perhaps the last thing they care about is the food they are eating. If you start talking about raw food or health, they may not be interested at all — because their other concerns are more pressing to them.

To be successful, you want to attract, not force. Imagine for a moment how a magnet works. Magnets can either attract (pull toward) or repel (push away) other magnets or metal objects. If you were holding two magnets, you could actually feel the force field between them, called magnetism. You can probably observe the same thing when you watch someone sharing information with another person — whether they are attracting that person's interest or repelling them.

If people feel like information is being forced upon them or the conversation is more of an argument, the message is lost. However, if you focus on being an example, you will find that people start coming to you.

Sometimes, we get so enthusiastic when we know something works that ego can creep in if people don't agree with what you are doing. You may have seen this out there with certain health experts who believe that their way is the only way. You know what's happening? They're talking because they want to be right. They're talking because they want people to look at them and say, "You're the guy who knows all the answers."

The truth is that no one knows ALL the answers. If you hear someone whose overall message sounds like "Me, me, me...this is my message and I'm going to get it out there," they are likely ego-centered instead of heart-centered. If we truly care about people, we can trust that they will be attracted to our information when they are ready. And if we share it in a heart-centered way, we can be more certain to pass on the message of health.

So here are some guidelines for successfully sharing the message of health:

- BE AN EXAMPLE. Don't tell people about it, just live the *High Raw* lifestyle and let people see your results.

- ATTRACT. Let people come to you. Understand their interests, needs and problems and start there. Do not force your message upon them if they have different interests, needs and problems.

- KEEP IT SIMPLE. Start simple when it comes to teaching others about *High Raw*. If people are overwhelmed, they are less likely to be enthusiastic about your message. Take your friends to a raw food restaurant and let them experience the food. That's pretty simple. My wife, Annmarie, and I do this when we are introducing people to raw food. Most people are pretty excited and say, "Wow, I didn't even know that this was what raw food could be." Even though you may not advocate heavy gourmet raw food on a regular basis, it can be an excellent bridge to show people how good raw food can be.

  Another example is to simply share a green powder drink with a family member. Have them add this drink each day...that's it. Once they get used to that and start feeling better, give them something else. Take it one step at a time and keep it simple.

- STAY HEART-CENTERED. If people aren't ready for your message, don't make it personal. Share the message of health to those who are ready.

We all want to get along and be accepted by our families, don't we? Yet one of the challenges with changing the way you eat is that your family will often have an opinion...and it may not be in your favor. A different way of eating is a change and people don't always like change, even if it's good.

People often resist change. The field of change management actually has tools and techniques to help people get through change. Change management experts help keep employees from sabotaging change in an organization, so that change can occur successfully. But we don't have a team of change management experts to help us with our family members...so it's important to realize that there may be some resistance when you change your diet and lifestyle.

Here are some tips for helping yourself and your family embrace your healthy lifestyle changes:

- BE A CHANGE AGENT. Change agents are people selected in organizations to help a change effort be successful. Interestingly, change agents pretty much do exactly what I outlined in the section above, on spreading your *High Raw* message. When you keep in mind that you are attracting the interest of your family members, rather than forcing your new opinions or behaviors, it can be a lot easier on everyone.

- LET GO. When you can let go of seeking your family member's approval and trust that what you are doing makes you feel good, it's easier to calmly stick to your new habits.

- GO AT YOUR OWN PACE. When you start your health journey at your own pace, you will feel less stressed and more energized about the changes you are making. This will actually have a positive effect on your family members.

If they see you overwhelmed and stressed, they will be less likely to think what you are doing is beneficial. In other words, what's better for you is better for them — that's a bonus!

- **SHARE INFORMATION WHEN THEY ASK.** Your family members may ask you why you are doing what you're doing. They may want to see more information. Have some resources to share with them. Start with a simple article or perhaps, a simple book that gives them a good overview without being too technical.

- **RELEASE JUDGMENT.** Sometimes family members don't want to embrace what you are doing because either they are judging you or they feel you are judging them. If you equally embrace everyone's ability to do what they feel is right for them, your family members will feel it. No one likes to be judged. You may find that when your family members see that you are not judging them, they won't judge you either.

TAKING IT ON THE ROAD — AT WORK AND ON VACATION

It's important for you to live your life, which means that sometimes you will be on vacation, at a work event, or in a situation (like during the holidays) where you might divert from your healthy eating habits. People always ask me, "Every so often I vacation from a raw, healthy lifestyle and eat cooked foods, let's say at my mom's house. Am I wasting all my previous efforts?" No. Some people will tell you that you are wasting your previous efforts, but I don't believe it.

Remember, with the *High Raw* lifestyle, your goal is not to be 100% perfect. Your goal is to always be moving toward optimal health. If you get off track, recognize that you are and get back on again. If you judge yourself, you will only end up feeling bad, which only serves to make matters worse.

The good news is, once you've created the habit of a *High Raw* lifestyle, you know how to get back if you've gotten off track. You might not feel good after eating some processed foods, but trust that you can feel better tomorrow when you reinstate your healthy habits.

Over time, you may come up with some strategies to help you eat healthy, even when traveling, at work or during the holidays. Perhaps you will plan ahead and bring healthy food with you or choose a restaurant where you can get the meal you want. But in life, there are times when even the best planning goes awry. The key is not to make your healthy lifestyle one of worry and stress. When you trust that you are doing your best, you'll enjoy the journey that much more.

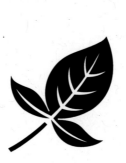

CHAPTER 18

BECOMING CONSCIOUS BEINGS

CLEANSING YOURSELF, CLEANSING THE PLANET

Something interesting happens when you start to follow a healthy *High Raw* lifestyle. First of all, when you eat a largely plant-based diet, full of ripe, raw vegetables, fruits, nuts and seeds, you begin to cleanse your body. As you focus on lifestyle changes, like drinking pure water, taking full, deep breaths, exercising and reducing stress, you also begin to cleanse your mind.

If you pay attention, you may in fact notice that you feel more connected in mind and body. From this place, instead of focusing on needing a quick fix to get through busy times, you begin to build sustainable energy, sustainable health. What does this mean? Sustainable means that you consciously use resources in the present moment, with an eye toward having plenty of reserves for the future. We understand this concept when it comes to the environment, but what about YOUR energy and health reserves? Are you willing to use up your own health and energy now — and have nothing left for a happy, vital future?

When you make a commitment to follow a healthy *High Raw* lifestyle, you are making a commitment to the present

AND future of your energy and health. The amazing thing is that as you start building sustainable health for yourself — as you start to feel connected in mind and body — you often find that you start to feel more connected to your community and to the planet. You begin to seek out ways to build sustainability all around you.

I'm not sure why this happens, but cleansing yourself often leads to cleansing the planet. It may start out by producing less trash from packaged foods and progress to saving precious resources through eating less meat and eventually, using sustainable energy sources.

The thing is, I think when we experience optimal health, we want to share it with others. We want everyone — people, animals, the planet — to feel as good as we do. It's possible that as one person heals, it makes a bigger impact on world health than any of us can imagine.

ACHIEVING OPTIMAL HEALTH

So what is optimal health? Is it something we reach and then we're done — kind of like making it to the top of the mountain? Do you think achieving optimal health is like hiking up Mt. Everest, with major challenges along a steep, frozen, uphill path and a quick celebration at the top? What if achieving optimal health were more like a moderately strenuous, yet enjoyable trek through the rainforest, with some ups and some downs, some flat spots — and of course, some incredible views all along the way?

In my mind, you never get "there" when it comes to optimal health. It's not a place to stop, where everything is simply done. Instead, it's a lifestyle of habits. It has its ups, its downs, its plateaus and its peaks. Most of all, it's meant to be a gentle journey, not one of worry and suffering, but one of discovery and enlightenment.

The real goal is to keep it simple — to stick to the basics and to have fun. The Five Principles of High Raw are guidelines for you to follow at your own pace. They represent the basics of healthy living in a world that perhaps, has gotten a bit off track in some places. At first, you may feel like you have to go out of your way to develop and stick to your healthy habits, but as you build sustainable energy and health, you will find that everything becomes easier. You may even feel like you are awakening, blossoming, coming alive.

RADIATING A HEALTHY NEW ENERGY

The new High Raw paradigm of health is that optimal health can be easy. *The Five Principles of High Raw* are your foundation — something you can stand on, guidelines to evaluate questions, a place to return to if you've gone off track. And it is something you do your way — because when you've gone through the Five Principles of High Raw, you understand and honor what your body needs.

We no longer have to be concerned about numbers and percentages of raw. I don't think percentage matters at all. A percentage is just about our need to be certain about something, like the glycemic index of potatoes. Our life is not about numbers. If it were, 7's would be growing off trees and 124's would be sprouting from the soil instead of fruits and vegetables. High Raw, to me, is not about food...it's about being centered. It's about feeling good and having energy. It's about taking care of me. It's about being kind to other creatures. It's about being conscious of the environment and the land we live on and with. Most importantly, High Raw about spreading a gentle message through example to a much larger group of people who may have lost touch with their own inner nature. They may be feeling down, or sick or unhappy. And they may no longer consciously recognize how good real, live food can make you feel.

NOW IT'S YOUR TURN....

As we improve our health we all become more conscious beings. We clean up our internal sludge and we're able to radiate a different energy...this is the kind of energy that will save the planet. That's the High Raw lifestyle. If you take the Five Principles of High Raw, you're going to be OK. What's going to happen is that you're going to radiate a sustainable energy — the kind of energy that keeps you feeling your best — and the kind of energy that others can see. You will no longer need to explain to people what you are doing because the glow of good health will speak for itself.

So I invite you to finish this book for yourself. Because YOU have the answers that you truly need. In the space below, write the answer to the following question: What is one action that you can take right now based on what you've learned in this book?

NOTES

Chapter 1

1 *Primary Health Care: Now More Than Ever*. The World Health Report 2008, p. 32.

2 Fallon, Sally. "Nasty, Brutish, and Short? Part1," Weed Wanderings With Sun Weed, June 2005.

Chapter 2

1 Roychoudhuri, Onnesha. *Michael Pollan Debunks Food Myths*, February 22, 2008. http://www.michaelpollan.com/press.php?id=92

2 ibid.

3 Adams, D. "Journals Aim to Curb Drug Industry Sway Over Studies," *American Medical News*, September 3, 2001.

4 ibid.

5 Adams, Mike. "Scientific medical journals like JAMA fail basic credibility standards; medical journals become increasingly irrelevant," *Natural News*, August 19, 2004.

6 Stanford School of Medicine Press Release. "New Stanford medical center policy limits drug company access and gifts," September 12, 2006.

7 ibid.

8 Staff Reporter. "US Congress told use of BPA in formula cans safe," *NutraIngredients.com*, January 5, 2009.

9 Martin, Andrew. "Fighting on a Battlefield the Size of a Milk Label," The New York Times, March 9, 2008.

10 Farm Animal Statistics: Meat Consumption. The Humane Society of the United States, November 30, 2006. http://www.hsus.org/farm/resources/pubs/stats_meat_consumption.html

11 Brown, Lester, R. Plan B 2.0: Rescuing a Planet Under Stress and a Civilization in Trouble, W. W. Norton; Exp Upd edition, 2006, p. 81.

12 ibid, p. 170.

13 Kranish, Michael. "Flaws are found in validating medical studies," *Boston Globe*, August 15, 2005.

14 Newport, Frank. "Americans Get Plenty of Health News on TV, but Tend Not to Trust It," September, 22, 2002, Gallup.com. http://www.gallup.com/poll/6883/Americans-Get-Plenty-Health-News-TV-Tend-Trust.aspx

15 Brownfield, Erica, D., et. al., "Direct-to-Consumer Drug Advertisements on Network Television: An Exploration of Quantity, Frequency and Placement," *Journal of Health Communication*, Volume 9: 491 – 497, 2004.

16 "2006 Drunk Driving Statistics," Alcohol Alert. http://www.alcoholalert.com/drunk-driving-statistics.html

17 Null, Gary, PhD., et. al. "Death By Medicine," *Life Extension Magazine*, March 2004, p. 3.

18 Russell, Christine, "Science Reporting by Press Release," *Columbia Journalism Review*, The Observatory, November 14, 62008. http://www.cjr.org/the_observatory/science_reporting_by_press_rel.php?page=2

19 Reuters. "Coffee: Top Source of Antioxidants," *Fox News*, August 28, 2005. http://www.foxnews.com/story/0,2933,167269,00.html

Chapter 3

1 Cousens, Gabriel, MD, *Rainbow Green Live Food Cuisine*, (Berkley: North Atlantic Books, 2003), p. 109.

2 Campbell, Colin, T., Ph.D., Campbell, Thomas M. II, The China Study: *The Most Comprehensive Study of Nutrition Ever Conducted and the Startling Implications for Diet, Weight Loss and Long-term Health*, (Dallas: Benbella Books, 2006), p. 5.

3 ibid, pp. 22 – 24.

4 Robbins, John, *Diet for a New America*, (HJ Kramer, 1998), p. 367.

5 Robbins, John, *The Food Revolution: How Your Diet Can Help Save Your Life and Our World*, (Berkeley: Conari Press, 2001), p. 258.

6 Robbins, John, *Diet for a New America*, (HJ Kramer, 1998), p. 365.

7 Robbins, John, *The Food Revolution: How Your Diet Can Help Save Your Life and Our World*, (Berkeley: Conari Press, 2001), p. 266.

Chapter 7

1 Grier, Tom, MS, "Will There Ever Be An Accurate Test for Lyme Disease?" CanLyme, Canadian Lyme Disease Foundation, January 19, 2009. http://www.canlyme.com/flawedtest.html

2 Bacon, Rendi Murphree, MS, Kugeler, Kiersten J., MPH, Mead, Paul S. MD, "Surveillance for Lyme Disease — United States, 1992–2006," Centers for Disease Control and Prevention Division of Vector-Borne Infectious Diseases, National Center for Zoonotic Vector-Borne and Enteric Diseases, http://www.cdc.gov/mmwr/preview/mmwrhtml/ss5710a1.htm

3 Pacholok, Sally M., R.N. and Stuart, Jeffrey, J., D.O., *Could it Be B12?: An Epidemic of Misdiagnosis*, (Sanger: Quill Driver Books/World Dancer Press, Inc., 2005), p. 10.

3 "Sex Differences in Cardio/Cerebovascular Diseases," Society for Women's Health Research. http://www.womenshealthresearch.org/site/PageServer?pagename=hs_facts_cardio

Chapter 10

1 Maltz, Maxwell, M.D., F.I.C.S., *The New Psycho-Cybernetics*, (New York: Penguin Putnam Books, 2001).

Chapter 12

1 "Pharmaceuticals and Personal Care Products in Water," US Environmental Protection Agency. http://www.epa.gov/waterscience/ppcp/

2 Batmanghelidj, Fereydoon, M.D., *Your Body's Many Cries For Water*, (Vienna: Global Health Solutions, Inc., 1997).

3 "Dehydration," MayoClinic.com. http://www.mayoclinic.com/health/dehydration/DS00561/DSECTION=symptoms

Chapter 15

1 "Enzymes and Longevity," *University of Natural Healing, Inc.*, 1991. http://www.living-foods.com/articles/enzymes.html

2 Pacholok, Sally M., R.N. and Stuart, Jeffrey J., D.O., *Could It Be B12?* (Sanger: Quill Driver Books, 2005), pp. 4 – 5.

3 ibid., pp. 13 – 15.

4 Adams, Mike, "Vitamin D myths, facts, and statistics," NewsTarget.com, 1 Jan 2005. http://www.newstarget.com/003069.html

5 Pick, Marcelle, OB/GYN NP, "Is vitamin D deficiency casting a cloud over your health?" *Women to Women*, June 27, 2005. http://www.womentowomen.com/nutritionandweightloss/vitamind.aspx

6 Blake, Paul, "Scientifically Tested Olive Leaf Herb Is Known To Kill Every Virus And Germ Known To Man," *ChattanoogaHealth.com*, May 27, 2008. http://www.chattanoogahealth.com/articles/557/1/Scientifically-Tested-Olive-Leaf-Herb-Is-Known-To-Kill-Every-Virus-And-Germ-Known-To-Man/Page1.html

7 Ehrlich, Steven D., N.M.D., ed., "Cat's claw," University of Maryland Medical Center, February, 24, 2007. http://www.umm.edu/altmed/articles/cats-claw-000229.htm

8 ibid.

BIBLIOGRAPHY

"2006 Drunk Driving Statistics," Alcohol Alert

Adams, D. "Journals Aim to Curb Drug Industry Sway Over Studies," *American Medical News*, September 3, 2001

Adams, Mike. "Scientific medical journals like JAMA fail basic credibility standards; medical journals become increasingly irrelevant," *Natural News*, August 19, 2004

Adams, Mike, "Vitamin D myths, facts, and statistics," *NewsTarget.com*, 1 Jan 2005

Bacon, Rendi Murphree, MS, Kugeler, Kiersten J., MPH, Mead, Paul S. M.D. "Surveillance for Lyme Disease — United States, 1992–2006," Centers for Disease Control and Prevention Division of Vector-Borne Infectious Diseases, National Center for Zoonotic Vector–Borne and Enteric Diseases

Batmanghelidj, Fereydoon, M.D. *Your Body's Many Cries For Water*, Vienna: Global Health Solutions, Inc., 1997.

Blake, Paul, "Scientifically Tested Olive Leaf Herb Is Known To Kill Every Virus And Germ Known To Man," *ChattanoogaHealth.com*, May 27, 2008

Brown, Lester, R. *Plan B 2.0: Rescuing a Planet Under Stress and a Civilization in Trouble*, Expanded updated edition, New York: W. W. Norton & Company, 2006.

Brownfield, Erica, D., et. al. "Direct-to-Consumer Drug Advertisements on Network Television: An Exploration of Quantity, Frequency and Placement," *Journal of Health Communication* 9 (2004): 491 – 497.

Boutenko, Victoria. *Green for Life*, Ashland: Raw Family Publishing, 2005.

Buhner, Stephen Harrod. *Healing Lyme: Natural Healing And Prevention of Lyme Borreliosis And Its Coinfections*, San Diego: Raven Press, 2005.

Campbell, Colin, T., Ph.D. Campbell, Thomas M. II, *The China Study: The Most Comprehensive Study of Nutrition Ever Conducted and the Startling Implications for Diet, Weight Loss and Long-term Health*, Dallas: Benbella Books, 2006.

Cousens, Gabriel, M.D. *Rainbow Green Live Food Cuisine*, Berkley: North Atlantic Books, 2003.

Covey, Steven R. *The Seven Habits of Highly Effective People*, New York: Free Press, 1989.

"Dehydration," *MayoClinic.com*

"Enzymes and Longevity," *University of Natural Healing, Inc.*, 1991

Ehrlich, Steven D., N.M.D., ed., "Cat's claw," University of Maryland Medical Center, February, 24, 2007

Fackelmann, Kathleen. "Stress can ravage the body, unless the mind says no: A positive outlook can reduce impact of stress on health," USA Today, March 22, 2005

Fallon, Sally. "Nasty, Brutish, and Short? Part1," Weed Wanderings With Sun Weed, June 2005

Farm Animal Statistics: *Meat Consumption*. The Humane Society of the United States, November 30, 2006

Graham, Douglas, N., D.C. *The 80/10/10 Diet*, Key Largo: FoodnSport Press, 2006.

Grier, Tom, MS. "Will There Ever Be An Accurate Test for Lyme Disease?" CanLyme, Canadian Lyme Disease Foundation, January 19, 2009

Hill, Napoleon. *Think and Grow Rich: Revised and Updated for the 21st Century*, New York: Penguin, 2005.

Hyman, Mark, M.D. *The UltraMind Solution: Fix Your Broken Brain by Healing Your Body First*, New York: Scribner, 2009.

Hyman, Mark, M.D. and Liponis, Mark. *Ultraprevention: The 6-Week Plan That Will Make You Healthy for Life*, New York: Atria Books, 2003.